Homeopathy

Everything You Need to Get Started With Confidence

(The Complete Guide to Homeopathic Medicine and Treatment of Common Disorders)

Oscar Cozad

Published By **Region Loviusher**

Oscar Cozad

All Rights Reserved

Homeopathy: Everything You Need to Get Started With Confidence (The Complete Guide to Homeopathic Medicine and Treatment of Common Disorders)

ISBN   978-1-998038-44-2

No part of this guidebook shall be reproduced in any form without permission in writing from the publisher except in the case of brief quotations embodied in critical articles or reviews.

Legal & Disclaimer

The information contained in this book is not designed to replace or take the place of any form of medicine or professional medical advice. The information in this book has been provided for educational & entertainment purposes only.

The information contained in this book has been compiled from sources deemed reliable, and it is accurate to the best of the Author's knowledge; however, the Author cannot guarantee its accuracy and validity and cannot be held liable for any errors or omissions. Changes are periodically made to this book. You must consult your doctor or get professional medical advice before using any of the suggested remedies, techniques, or information in this book.

Table Of Contents

Chapter 1: What it Is

We must start with the things that aren't.

If I inform people that I'm an herbalist, there's always an instant when the situation changes. Sometimes, it's a distancing. block me off due to having heard something regardless of how inaccurate or incomplete they believe that it was a hoax. When they don't distancing the two, there's a flash of connecting: they claim to have had the experience, or that someone knows has used it believed it to be remarkable. However, in the end the reality is that they believe they are aware of what it is, yet they aren't sure. The term "homeopathy" has come into usage with an incorrect definition.

It's a good thing that we even have people who recognize the term. The word is not widely known, and any mention of it helps to raise awareness about its existence.

However, when it is used in the context of its commonly misinterpreted definition of a broad phrase that encompasses every alternative treatment, or any other treatment that is not conventional, or even anything "natural" - misunderstandings begin which can result in ill-informed decisions and conclusions.

Homeopathy is an important alternative to the field of complementary medical treatment. It's not herbal and nutrition, flower essences vitamins supplementation, diet vital oils, chiropractic or the practice of acupuncture. There are its own ways of doing things and products, as well as manufacturers as well as training courses as well as books as well as professional and consumer organizations and standards for certification. One thing that it shares with the practices it's usually classified with is that it's not a conventional treatment.

The misunderstanding can cause many different problems that go that go beyond a casual conversation. If someone claims to their friend that they've seen great results using homeopathy and they go seeking out what they perceive as a "homeopath" or a "homeopathic doctor," they could have a different experience or may not be able to get the results they're hoping for. In the event that news outlets make use of the word "homeopathic medicine" incorrectly, the stigma of homeopathy comes due to the wrongdoing of many people without any connection to the practice. When a consumer advocate is trying to inform a lobbyist, or legislator, they might talk past one another to the point that there is no progress. That's not to suggest that other strategies do not have flaws and they are efficient, however in order to choose the best tool for any assignment, we must understand what the actual tools are.

The homeopathic approach is similar to the different "natural" modalities in that it utilizes medicines found in the natural world. Every modality comes with its own set of principles on using the ingredients of nature. And each alters natural resources according to its own unique way. Herbal medicine, for instance could dry out a plant to form the basis for tea, then powder the tea to make capsules, or even make it a liquid and then soak it in order to make an tincture. Homeopathic medicine is made from organic sources, modified to create a way which are only used within the field of homeopathy. The process is explained in Chapter 3.

The diagram below will show how homeopathy differs from different therapies. "Homeopathic" is not a term used to describe "alternative" or "natural." Homeopathy is a individual kind of healing that is natural.

Classical Homeopathy

The best method to understand homeopathy is to tell the narrative of the beginning.

In 1790, Germany in 1790, a physician translated a textbook for medical students on the various medicines available that day, and included theories on how they functioned. Certain theories struck the doctor as absurd when reached the chapter of quinine, the doctor been through with his research.

Everybody recognized quinine as a potent treatment for malaria. It was which was then known by the name of intermittent fever. It was the translator Samuel Hahnemann, had benefitted from it many years ago when he had malaria. However, the author of the textbook said que quinine was effective due to it's "fortifying effect on the stomach," that Hahnemann had not experienced, and that did not make sense given the many other substances just as bitter, strong, as well as "fortifying" as quinine but they didn't cure malaria.

Being a doctor and researcher Hahnemann sought information. "By way of experiment," Hahnemann wrote in his journal, he bought some quinine, and began taking the doses in a measured amount daily, just as would have administered to patients suffering from malaria. Then, within a short time, he started to show signs even though he was a healthy patient taking medicine and, in essence, it was a deliberate poisoning of himself. He became weak and tired His heart beat a lot faster and his cheeks became pink; he was shivering, could not think and was very anxious. In addition, his bones were as if they were numb and heavy. It was a surprise to discover the symptoms were common when he contracted malaria. When he took an amount of quinine, the symptoms would be similar for several hours then when he stopped the dose it was back to normal. The malaria wasn't actually present because of quinine. He'd been able to get a fake, temporary model of malaria. Incredulous that he had proved that the writer of the textbook was to be wrong, by locating a new explanation, he took an annotation in his own translation: "Substances which excite a kind of fever extinguish the types of intermittent fever."

Hahnemann was about to make the most significant discovery which his study was later to confirm was widely reported throughout the history of. He took years to fully comprehend it however, when he finally did the research, he formulated it using Latin: "Similia similibus curentur," literally "Let likes be cured by the things that are most like them" and eventually was shortened in "Like cures like" or the Law of Similars. It is the first distinctive feature of homeopathy and is named in honor of the Greek meaning "same" and "suffering." Homeopathy alleviates the suffering of patients who suffer from illness with the help of a drug which causes the same signs in healthy people.

Hahnemann was an ardent researcher. When his experiments and studies proved his findings of the Law of Similars, he created it into a complete medical approach. The same way the research on quinine had been conducted and other drugs, he also tested various medicines and minerals, including plants as well as animal substances to discover what signs as "artificial diseases" they produced for healthy individuals Then he utilized these to tackle those issues within his clinic. Clinical experience proved that using the Law of Similars was a reliable method to aid patients.

Through his day-long experiment using quinine Hahnemann developed not just an innovative method of practicing but also a brand new method to study the effects of the drugs. In the future, he would write that, if you were trying to learn about a particular medicine is not logical to try it on patients who were sick, since then it is difficult to discern the drug's actions in their entirety - instead, you observe it in conjunction with the signs of disease. A controlled application of a medication to people who are healthy to see the effects it has on them is referred to as proving. It remains the standard in the way we study the benefits of homeopathic medicine. Today, tests must be done with only people who are healthy, well informed and willing adult individuals, and never with individuals or animals that have been ill or impaired or compromised in some way.

There was an additional breakthrough to be discovered. A lot of medicines can be toxic when taken when taken in large quantities, and Hahnemann tried small and less of them to find out how much required to create the cure. This was in contrast to practices used in conventional "heroic medicine" of the times, when medications were administered as high as the tolerance limits of a patient. "Bleeding" patients by bloodletting and "sweating" them or "purging" the patient with vomiting or diarrhea were considered as a way to get rid from illness. Hahnemann believed that this kind of treatment was inefficient and depleting patients who required strength to recover. In search of the most effective dosage He diluted his medication by vigorously shaking them during the dilution process to see if they were still effective. And, even more to his delight, they performed better in fully.

In the wake of the Law of Similars as the initial defining element of homeopathy, the minimal dose, and in particular this way for making medicine became the second. Hahnemann identified it as "dynamization" but "potentization" has now become a more popular word. Potentized medications are created through several steps that involve shaking and dilution. The amount of dilution as well as the quantity of steps produce different strengths of the medicine.

Another aspect of homeopathy that Hahnemann advocated was the practice of using a individual medicine at a given period of. Hahnemann believed that when different the medicines are mixed and mixed together, it is not just difficult to discern which one is working, but also they could also interfere in a way. Additionally, his studies have shown that all medicines produced symptoms that affected the entire human body, with physical emotional, and mental symptoms being a result of the same drug. If he was able to identify the correct remedy for the entire person this one remedy could assist them on all levels of their lives. One treatment at a moment is a third characteristic of homeopathy in the classical technique developed by Hahnemann.

Hahnemann was a homeopath who practiced throughout his lifetime, constantly developing it in accordance with his experiences in the clinic, while affirming the fundamentals. The doctors who studied under his practice took homeopathy into other countries. Although there have been many fluctuations and fluctuations over the years, it has continued to be utilized throughout the globe.

From Then to Now

Students of Hahnemann propagated homeopathy throughout Europe as well as to his home in the United States even during his period of time. Within the U.S. the homeopathic medical colleges and professional societies rapidly expanded across the nation. They were the American Institute of Homeopathy (AIH) is the first medical society of the national U.S., was founded in 1844, long prior to that of the American Medical Association (AMA). The homeopathic method proved to be extremely effective in the terrible epidemics of the nineteenth century like yellow fever and cholera. It also aiding in the fight against yellow fever and cholera on Civil War battlefields, and was adopted by citizens of all kinds of backgrounds, ranging from rural people to elites in the city. At the beginning of the century, it could be difficult to know what type of medicine were more popular in the years to come, given that they were both well-known and established.

However, by 1920 homeopathy was in the receding into the background. Internal divisions had weakened the practice, and changing social views led to adjustments regarding health medical care. Regulations that were introduced in the 1990s slowed hospitals that were homeopathic, resulting in there was a decline in doctors receiving instruction in homeopathy. The homeopathic profession was in decline within the U.S. for half a century.

In the 1970s, certain physicians as well as consumers were seeking a different way of doing medicine, and they found the answer in an old method called homeopathy. Homeopathy was given the name of National Center for Homeopathy was established in 1974 as a means to encourage homeopathy by education. The training programs began to pop into existence, which led to the creation of the system of accreditation for schools and practitioner accreditation that protects the practice and all who profit from the benefits of it. Homeopathy today is more varied and easily available than it was when it was in its glory just over 100 years earlier.

The Samuel Hahnemann monument on Scott Circle in Washington, D.C. demonstrates the importance of homeopathy throughout American the past. The monument was inaugurated on the 21st of June in 1900, by the president William McKinley. A large number of people attended the dedication ceremony. The United States Marine Band played.

The monument was dedicated on the 21st of June of 2000. It was then re-dedicated by a consortium of professional and consumer organizations that was led by the American Institute of Homeopathy, the same body that started the construction of the monument over one hundred years prior. The statue that is larger than life of Hahnemann is surrounded by friezes that depict significant events of his work. The statue is still an impressive and insightful tribute of Hahnemann as well as homeopathy.

Other Types of Homeopathy

The experiments of Hahnemann led him to create classical homeopathy that continues to be practiced in similar to the way it is today. I'm a classical homopath and this is a book about homeopathy that was classical and, therefore, as is the norm in this area by saying "homeopathy" I mean the traditional method of treating one patient at one time. There are different approaches came up with after the time of Hahnemann in order to adjust homeopathy so that it can be more in line to Western standards of medicine.

Classical homeopathy is an effective solid, secure, and reliable therapy method that is employed to treat almost everything, however it requires some training before you can use it properly. The process of learning the system in its entirety is a bit difficult; expert professionals study for a long time. People at home are able to get started with a little education, however dealing with minor illnesses requires much more expertise than simply walking into the drugstore to buy items off the shelves as we're accustomed to do. In order to create a solution which doesn't need any education or experience, companies create combinations of treatments.

Many health food stores stock one-off remedies, the majority of the medicines that are sold to the public today are mixture treatments. These are formulations that comprise several potentized single medications mixed. These formulas can be used in order for relieving the discomfort caused by menstrual period pain, teething and arthritis, as well as muscles strains, headaches and many more. These are developed by companies who mix a limited number of remedies frequently used to treat these ailments. Because there are a myriad of solutions that could be used to treat a specific issue, manufacturers will pick different categories of remedies in their formulations.

Store shelves are stocked with combinations of remedies

The sales records of their products prove it the combination remedy are extremely effective because the packaging and labels are similar to those used in generic (OTC) remedies They can provide an ideal way to test the homeopathic method a go. It is also extremely affordable and suitable to treat people of all ages and ailments. The FDA supervises their manufacturing and labeling in the same way as they regulate individual remedies.

Homeopathy is a science that teaches us that there is only one remedy for everyone who is sick and therefore, combination treatments can effectively be described as an investment in hedges. If a combination remedy works most likely due to that one of the remedies that they have is the best for the patient while the other remedies have none of any effect. Most of the remedies in combination treatments are lower potency, meaning they won't have any effect in the absence of being the right option for the particular situation. Combination remedies are extremely secure when they are used in accordance with instructions from the manufacturer. Additionally, access and convenience can be crucial for many people.

A disadvantage of combining remedies is that, if they do not make a difference, someone who is new to the practice might conclude that all the homeopathic remedies are bogus. Naturally, we would not reach the same conclusion regarding all traditional medicine if we used any over-the-counter painkiller and feeling the pain, but that's another subject for a different time. In reality, if an ointment or combination doesn't yield outcomes, it's probably because there is a need for a natural medication that the manufacturer could not find in the formulation. If a mixture remedy is effective however it stops the reason could be that an alternative remedy or higher potency is required. Classical homeopathy, at home or in conjunction with an expert, may be used when homeopathy in combination does not suffice.

One of the disadvantages of combination therapies is that they're not tailored to each individual in the way that Hahnemann's classic approach would require. So, while they might ease symptoms for a short time but they're not usually sufficient to help in the restoration of health for those suffering from chronic ailments. In this case, the help of the classically trained homeopath may provide more benefit for the longer term.

Additionally, there are non-classical practitioners that use combinations of remedies typically in the form of liquid drops used several times throughout the every day. They typically use professional formulations that are more potent than those available at stores and could offer a variety of options at once. There are also professionals who utilize devices for "test" for what remedy is required, and possibly use them to "make" potentized remedies by exposure of sugar pellets to electrical frequencies. There are manufacturers who provide the homeopathic "injectables" for use by health professionals who are licensed in a practice area that is quite different from the fundamental principles of homeopathy.

Professional homeopathy is not a regulated form of homeopathy compared to classical homeopathy. Training as well as "certification" are administered mostly by the makers of the drugs, not by accredited homeopathy colleges and programs for training. Additionally, patients usually purchases these combination medicines through the doctor, which creates an incentive to overprescribe. The majority of a doctor's earnings could be derived from the products they offer to clients and patients. Because of this, traditional homeopaths are generally cautious of mix prescribers as some believe that this practice is detrimental to the efforts of homeopathy to be recognized as a field of study.

Once you've realized how something that seems difficult as homeopathy is actually possible you'll be able to accept any thing without paying it close consideration.

Part II contains stories about patients who were helped by traditional homeopathy. I'd like to also share my experience of being introduced to the potential of combining remedies.

Julia: Uterine Cancer

Twenty years ago, while mingling in a small group of parents at the dance class where our children were enrolled in classes I had a conversation with a woman that appeared attractive and bright. I could tell she was from large family members because I'd previously seen her with a minimum of five kids from different ages. Her eyes lit up when I mentioned that"I'm studying homeopathy." "Oh, homeopathy saved my life!"

I was preparing for that awkward moment in which she would reveal that with "homeopathy" she meant flower essences or herbs or energy healing. I had to make a decision on which of us to inform her that I was wrong and the time did not come. Instead, she shared an experience that will forever be one of the most important learning experiences.

10 years prior, Julia had been diagnosed with uterine cancer, which was pretty advanced by the time it was discovered. Julia was a mother of two children in that moment. The doctor told her that chemotherapy had a good probability of getting rid of the cancer. But she'd have to get her uterus surgically removed. No children. Being a mother was the reason she chose to continue living and, after some reflection with her husband, they considered other alternatives.

Julia altered her diet right away and she realized that would not be enough. An acquaintance had informed the story of a homeopath and she decided to visit. The doctor practiced homeopathy in combination and offered her "I don't even remember how many little dropper bottles" which she would use multiple times throughout the daily. There were timers throughout the house to ensure she was on a time. She visited the homeopath at least every month, and varied the dosage often. She also continued to have regular check-ups with her physician. Further tests gradually revealed that the cancer was decreasing. 18 months later, her doctor concluded that she did not have indication of disease. As she continued to undergo regular screenings according to her doctor's recommendations and she was able to have another six children and was cancer-free for the rest of her life. Recently, I learned from a friend of mine that she's now a fit and content mother of 12 with more to come.

It's clear that Julia's decision on how to deal with her condition was quite a bold decision that some may even consider that it was foolish. This was also atypical as a result of her choice as well as her ability to find a doctor who would be able to treat her since most homeopaths aren't willing to treat cancer patients, unless they're receiving conventional treatments. It's hard to comprehend the remedies that Julia's doctor recommended to her. Certainly, they were expert formulas superior to the ones available in shops - and even the techniques for selecting his remedies. However, I'm grateful to have her tale since it reminds me of the fact that there are many paths for success in homeopathy.

Chapter 2: Safety

The homeopathic method is among the most safe methods of health care. The medicines are not at risk of overdose, toxicity, drugs that interact or cause addiction. The drug can be utilized by those who are young, extremely old, delicate and pregnant in a way, and is just equally safe for people who are well-behaved. With a lifespan of more than 200 year olds, it's not anything new in this.

One of the major factors that determine the safety of homeopathy is the quality of the medicines. The majority part of chapter 3 is focused on this since they're hard to understand. Because they're dilute, there'd have no risk even if a person ate all of them, which is what kids are most likely to do, since the taste of the pellets is similar to sugar. Because of their diluting properties, there's no risk of allergic reactions or toxic effects as well as no risk of an being overdosed. It is possible to make poisons as homeopathic remedies, and be in a safe environment.

Furthermore, the potentized remedies of homeopathy are able to work at a different level of the body than traditional drugs are able to do. They're completely distinct from conventional forms of medication, and therefore they aren't able to interact with traditional drugs. However, the reverse could happen: some conventional medicines hinder the effectiveness of potentized remedies. However, you'll be able to guarantee that traditional medicines will function even if you're practicing homeopathy.

Within the U.S. the Food and Drug Administration (FDA) supervises drug companies that are homeopathic just as they supervise conventional ones. Companies must follow FDA-required requirements for quality and safety in order to make sure that their products are well-balanced, safe and properly listed. There is no reason not to be sure when you purchase a natural medication as buying an over-the-counter cold or painkiller.

What you need to do to ensure security when using homeopathy is applying the same common sense as you do with other treatment at home. In the event of an emergency visit an ambulance. If that doesn't work then try something different. If the problem is getting worse or you're feeling like you're in a bind, quit looking for a solution at home, and seek expert help. Examine things objectively, remain focused and you'll be fine. Chapter 6 contains more specifics on safety as well as the effectiveness of home health care.

If you opt to visit an expert, which is recommended in the case of chronic or persistent ailments, they'll use the same type of extremely-dilute drugs that are FDA-regulated. They can be available over the counter but they'll utilize the same methods that are appropriate for medical treatment.

The medical field is structured at the professional level and therefore, there is a consistent set of qualifications that you should be looking for. Additionally, there is a way to evaluate the doctor's education background in addition. Refer to chapter 6 for further details.

One of the most sensible safety complaints I've come across regarding homeopathy is that it could delay receiving more suitable medical attention if it does not work. This is the case with any other type of self-care. It's a matter of not getting care due to any reason and getting a prescribed medicine from your doctor that doesn't be effective for your needs. That's not a genuine criticism of homeopathy. It is best to use good judgment and relying on the most reliable facts you can locate.

Chapter 3: Medicines

The expressions "medicines" and "remedies" can be used interchangeably within homeopathy. "Remedy" evokes the history of homeopathy. The practice has existed for since the beginning of time, making some its terms seem old-fashioned. "Medicine" is accurate to the extent it refers to something that you consume however its meanings aren't quite right. Nowadays "medicine" usually means a chemical, but is not the case with homeopathic remedies. As both words come with pluses and drawbacks they've been scattered in the pages of this book.

All homeopathic remedies start with a natural substance, and all are made through making potentization by diluting, then shaking, then diluting and shaking and repeating the process repeatedly. The only method of homeopathy which makes use of this method for the production of remedies. Different variations result from the sources of ingredients are utilized and how they are diluted and the number of steps that are utilized. Three variables indicate that one process can yield a vast array of medications. At present, there are more than three thousand remedies that are homeopathic.

Remedy Sources

They can be made of any substance - in fact everything. Hahnemann began with ingredients which were commonly used as drugs during his times. There are remedies made using sources employed in conventional and herbal medicines, like the chamomile (Chamomilla within homeopathy) and Ipecac (Ipecacuanha).

In the beginning, when Hahnemann's experiments began with conventional remedies that he was using Hahnemann and his fellow homeopaths added a variety of additional remedies of the animal, plant as well as mineral realms. A few examples of widely used plants are jasmine that is yellow (Gelsemium) as well as cedar (Thuja) as well as salvia (Salvia) Ruta (Ruta) as well as the devil's trumpet (Stramonium) as well as windflower (Pulsatilla). Animal remedies can include venoms derived of snakes like The bushmaster (Lachesis) insect species like honeybees (Apis) as well as pet products, such as dogs' milk (Lac caninum) as well as spiders like the Tarantula (Tarentula). Most mineral remedies originate taken from oyster shells (Calcarea carbonica), sea salt (Natrum muriaticum) and elements like Phosphorus (Phosphorus) along with Sulfur (Sulphur) as well as metals like Tin (Stannum) and copper (Cuprum) and silver (Argentum) as well as the gold (Aurum). A recent surge in interest in mysterious has given us some remedies created of "imponderables" like sunlight and moonlight. Researchers who are observing the trends of today's world have investigated Ozone and chocolate. With more than two hundred years of using homeopathy and homeopathy, we've only begun exploring all of the treatment resources the planet can offer.

Due to the potentization process, drugs can behave differently when used as natural remedies than in their natural nature. When using a herb, it's impossible to way to know how it'll behave when it's in potentized form until you perform a homeopathic test. There are many substances that have a variety of applications, sometimes even opposing ones when they're infused. A few remedies are derived from toxic substances, and the process of potentizing makes these substances totally safe and uncovering their hidden benefits. For instance, poison ivy is potent cure (Rhus toxicodendron) can help with certain skin issues, but has a powerful effect on a number of joint issues and has numerous remedies for chronic illness. While many of the remedies are derived from familiar sources, when they're made according to the homeopathic method, they're not as similar to their initial form, just in the same way that penicillin differs made from mold.

The homeopathic remedies are made using any natural source which includes the kingdom of plants, the animal kingdom, as well as mineral realm. On the next pages are a few typical remedies

Rhus toxicodendron is derived by poison Ivy. Plant remedies also comprise roots, leaves and even flowers from a vast assortment of species.

Lac caninum is a product made of the milk of dogs. Other sources of animal remedies comprise snake venoms, insect venoms and other animal products.

Aurum metallicum is a product of gold. The other mineral remedies comprise nonliving elements such as minerals, rocks, as well as other metals.

How They're Made

Hahnemann created himself his own remedies however, we'd be foolish to do such a labour-intensive tasks when we have machines that could do it quicker as well as more efficiently and in a safer manner. Modern remedies are produced through dedicated pharmaceutical manufacturers within factories which the FDA checks for quality and safety. Each remedy is created using the same method.

The manufacturing process starts by making the substance source into the form that is able to be dissolvable by water. It is simple for certain substances, including sea salt and substances that already have water-soluble liquids. In the case of other sources, there are distinct procedures that are appropriate for each. The document known as the Homeopathic Pharmacopoeia for the United States spells out the particulars, and is used by the manufacturers as well as the FDA to verify that each of the homeopathic medications are secure and reliable.

If there's a liquid type of the ingredient (a tincture) and the process of potentization starts. A measured amount of the tincture and water are mixed (dilution) and then agitated (succussion) over a number of stages. The resultant liquid is the potentized solution. Alcohol can be mixed with the water or to preserve the product. In order to make the remedy more convenient, it is typically supplied to the user as a pill such as lactose (milk sugar) or sucrose pellets, or tablets are filled with the cure, and then dried, and then bottled. The dried form doesn't degrade their medicinal properties as the ingredient is retained even after alcohol and water are gone. It's not a taste or alcohol. The taste is only sugar. Tablets and pellets are small and such a little amount is necessary to ensure that those who suffer from lactose intolerance or those with diabetes are able to use them without little or no problem. These potent remedies can be dispensed in ointments liquids and gels that can be applied topically.

The dilution percentage and quantity of steps define the efficacy of the solution and is identified with a number or the letter for example, 30X, or 12C. The amount is the number of times it was dispersed and succussed. The letters represent the dilution ratio. These letters represent Roman numbers. X stands for the number ten and C refers to 100. A remedy X has ten components during each stage of production (nine parts of water to one solution) and C remedies have 100 components (ninety-nine parts water for one solution). For instance an ingredient in the 30X potency is made by diluting 30 times in 9 parts water for one solution, and succussing between the diluting steps.

In the case of individual remedies, the manufacturing procedure is completed when the desired level of potency has been achieved. Combination remedies are created by mixing several previously potent single remedies.

This diagram outlines the initial three steps involved in creating an X-potency. Each step involves dilution, and succussion (agitation).

This same method is employed to create a C Potency however, with 99 parts of water per dilution.

This process is able to be carried on throughout the year to produce greater and more powerful substances.

The most difficult aspect to wrap our minds to is the notion it is true that "higher potencies," those which are generally thought of as stronger, are also the least dilute. 30C has a greater potency than 12X. Higher temperatures of 200C or more are considered extremely potent and should be used only by experts.

The potentization process is completed then the liquid that results drops onto sugar pellets, or tiny fast-dissolving sugar tablets to provide means of getting it to the user in a convenient way. Different sizes and shapes can be utilized; they serve as inert transporters of the medication and their shape does not affect the efficacy or safety of the treatment.

Tablets and sugar pellets utilized as carriers for the homeopathic medicine are very small and disintegrate easily when placed into the mouth.

Another type of remedy Hahnemann came up with at the end of his life which didn't become popular in the 20th century. in the present, it's extremely uncommon. The Fifty-Millesimal scale also known as the LM scale, which stands for short. which is the Roman numerals that represent fifty and 1,000. LM remedies are produced using a different method which requires more dilution as well as lower sucussion. They are dissolved in water, followed by shaking or stirring prior to every dose. These are only used within professional practices since the dose and timing need to be adjusted according to the particular patient's needs.

How They're Tested

As Hahnemann began to test medicines through provings in conjunction with his friends, family members, as well as other people and found that he had both similar patterns as well as individual differences in the effects they produced. He had recorded the effects of quinine for him in the first proving that I wrote about in Chapter 1. However, there were some who had different reactions. He realized that every remedy must be tested on a variety of individuals to discover its entire spectrum of actions. Most commonly-used remedies have been tested numerous times throughout the years and are considered "fully proved" only when the latest provings provide no facts.

Provings must always be conducted by well-informed, healthy, and adult participants who are willing to participate. This is essential in terms of ethics and since the evidence gathered from proof is as trustworthy in the hands of those who are writing about the findings. Modifications to thoughts, emotions physical and mental feelings are as crucial as what can be seen objectively which is why provers need to understand the details of what's going on in their bodies.

Provings are made using substances which are potent, therefore there is no risk that you'll get poisoned, toxic, or overdose. The remedies for only a short time that they begin to feel signs; they stop drinking the medicine at the point it begins taking effect. So, the effect of the treatment can be visible and can be eliminated rapidly.

For the most thorough provings each prover is assigned one supervisor who is qualified in homeopathy. Provers are regularly in contact with their supervisors over an extended duration because certain proving signs require a long time to manifest. Supervisors send the data on to the master prover who then compiles an report to the community of homeopathy. Proving documents are typically printed in the form of a book along with the details adding to the book of reference. In order to ensure objectivity, managers and provers aren't aware of the substance being proven until all the work is completed. Sometimes, even the chief proofer doesn't have a clue.

The only way to make it work is using solid and reliable data of evidence. Utilizing this Law of Similars entails matching the signs of a person's natural illness with the symptoms of the same "artificial disease" that's been identified in proofs. The wide range of natural ailments means that we require a large amount of specific information from provings to ensure an exact match. Once the evidence reveals every aspect of an "artificial disease" a remedy may cause, we are able to determine what natural signs it can alleviate. The list of symptoms that are associated with our most famous remedies stretch up to hundreds of pages in our book of reference. There is no one who suffers from all of these ailments and each one is only the smallest fraction of the remedies to be able of. That's why it's important to trying out each solution until no more signs are noticed.

Provings are the main source of knowledge about how each remedy works However, there are two other sources too. The poisonings of the body are one such source, since they're sort of accidental proof. There is plenty of historical facts about the accidental poisoning of substances later transformed into treatments. Medical diagnosis manuals today provide the signs of poisonings resulting from any toxic substance which are also created as non-toxic potentized remedies for homeopathy, ranging from snake bites to poisonous plants as well as heavy metals. The information provided is particularly helpful for homeopaths since provings cause minor symptoms and the remedies could prove useful in urgent instances that do not appear through provings, but rather are implied by poisonings. Naturally, a substance that is potentized is different from the substance in its original formulation, which is why we must conduct tests using the potentized solution to determine what is the "artificial disease" that it can cause, however often, poisonings indicate a different aspect of its effects.

The most reliable source of data is the clinical success which is, in essence the way that medicines function within the context of. This is where the homeopathic time of practice comes in useful. In some cases, a remedy may be provided based on the information obtained from tests and can cure another patient too. If it happens often enough the new application for the treatment is documented in the books on homeopathy, so it is available to doctors as they review the cases. Clinical success fills in the gaps which haven't been revealed through the tests. We have huge amounts of information on treatments which have been used for a long time. A few of the oldest remedies fill dozens of pages in book of reference for homeopathy, due to the clinical evidence that has identified their many advantages to a multitude of individuals throughout the ages.

How They're Sold

The remedies are available in health grocery stores, some pharmacies as well as online. One-time remedies are packaged in tiny bottles or tubes that are labelled with the source ingredient and usually the scientific name and the potency of the remedy, for instance "Arnica Montana 30C" or "Chamomilla 12X." Labels are also able to specify the use of the remedy that the FDA mandates for all drugs that are sold on the market. However, in the field of homeopathy, the indicated use is only a aspect of what a remedy could accomplish, as, in contrast to the usual prescription medications available, each remedy can be used for a variety of possibilities. In the event that a label would list all the benefits of Pulsatilla such as, say, it should be an entire 12 page booklet that is attached to each bottle. Single remedy manufacturers have to decide on one of the remedies' most frequent uses on the label.

Single remedies

Kits that are pre-assembled and contain only one remedy are a practical and economical way to get started on your own home remedy collection. They're available in many dimensions and strengths. They are sometimes targeted to specific reasons like emergency first aid, travel, baby care or animal health.

Kits for resolving problems

Because the FDA categorizes the majority of the homeopathic remedies available over the counter, everyone is able to purchase the medicines. Demand from customers is what draws the products into stores, however it is possible to not have them available in your local area. Stores that sell just one product have only the space they need and are flooded with options that they are unable to provide more than a limited choice. Phone and online orders allow you to easily access any remedy you want. It is beneficial to purchase from an online retailer that is specifically focused on homeopathic remedies as they have staff members that are knowledgeable and are willing to assist you with any your questions.

Natural sources of the homeopathic medicine and consistent manufacturing process make them extremely affordable since neither the source or the method are patented. If you purchase only one remedy, the price for shipping could surpass the value of the remedy in itself.

In the case of combination remedies the labels include an ingredient list generally between four to twelve and each one with a science-based name and the amount. It could be that there is a purpose of each ingredient, and the general application of the mix which is stated on the label. The combination remedies are becoming more readily offered in pharmacies, health food stores and grocery stores.

The name is derived from a mix remedy to treat insomnia

Chapter 4: Science

Referrals to "science" are often used in order to deny the validity of the notion of homeopathy. "It's not scientific." "There's no science behind it." Actually, those claims aren't accurate. There's a lot of scientific evidence that homeopathy uses for centuries as well as the most recent research conducted in clinical and lab situations. The section on Resources near the end of the book will direct you to a few of them.

One of the problems when studying homeopathy using the eyes of science is the fact that a lot of conventional tools and practices that are used in modern science don't work. In order to have the integrity of every investigation, it is essential select techniques that fit the subject matter we're investigating - it's not possible to, for instance utilize a microscope for examining the sound waves. If the wrong tools are employed to evaluate homeopathy, it will naturally end into appearing "unscientific" from a narrow and unfocused view of what science is supposed to be. When studies employ instruments that relate to the specifics of homeopathy, the science-based validity is evident.

The individual approach of Homeopathy as well as the potent remedies it offers require investigations which differ from methods used in normal medical research. But, the scientific approach can be considered an essential component of homeopathy. The definitions of science as method connect it to research as well as observations. They are referring to methods that are systematic and evidence, freedom from bias, and the quest for natural laws that can be tested as well as predictive data. Homeopathy ticks all these boxes with a vengeance. The practices mentioned are founded in the core of homeopathy. This includes everything from the method of making medicines and tested, all the way to how the treatment plans are developed and tested in clinical settings. Homeopathy, at its heart, is not a science at all.

The more reliable way of stating "It's not scientific" would be "It's not explainable by the conclusions that Science has drawn so far about the natural world." It isn't a reason to say there's something wrong regarding Science or even homeopathy; it's just a matter of working on opposite side of the road and a safe crosswalk isn't yet in place.

Clinical Trials

Its efficacy has been documented repeatedly by medical doctors and other practitioners However, it's a challenge to study using modern methods. Clinical trials are a standard procedure that require that researchers adhere to procedures designed for conventional medical practice, not specifically for homeopathy. The application of the standard design for homeopathy clinical trials is similar to trying to put bananas into an egg carton. The bananas just won't go in.

Take, for instance, one of the major components of drug research known as the randomized controlled trial (RCT). It is designed to avoid bias via standardization such as by assigning participants at random to one of two groups, an active or controlled group, which is a group that does not get the substance being investigated and instead is given an alternative that appears identical. The participants don't know what category they're in, and for double-blind studies, researchers don't even know. This is commonplace for homeopathy too In provings that are rigorous, participants are randomly placed in the active group which takes the medication or to a placebo group who takes pellets that are not medicated. Each group is followed exactly during the proving phase while supervisors do not know the group that is which until after the proving has been finished.

The standard drug research study the main question to be sought in conventional drug studies is "Does this medicine treat this condition effectively?" The RCT technique is used to examine the relation between a specific medication and a certain disease. The research design is in line with the questions being asked. You'll need to give the medication to those suffering from the illness and then observe the results.

When you practice homeopathy, it's not possible to inquire about that, as there isn't a specific medicine which treats a specific condition efficiently - rather, there's a medication that can treat every person. Five patients suffering from the same issue may require a variety of remedies homeopathically. Clinical trials that ask "does this homeopathic remedy treat this condition effectively?" or employing the same remedy for everyone in the active group is bound to fail.

We didn't realize about this and have decided to utilize a conventional RCT model for an experiment to determine the extent to which Arnica montana 30C can be beneficial for pains and aches during physical activity. It's a good idea to go to the Boston Marathon and engage participants who have just completed the race. They're divided into two groups: an active group as well as a control group. We offer Arnica 30C in the active group, and unmedicated sugar pellets to the group that controls. So far, everything is fine - it's the correct procedure to conduct an RCT.

The results are likely to be mixed. One thing is that we'll discover that Arnica 30C can help a specific, and probably tiny percentage of patients. It's because it's one of the many treatments available in this scenario. Certain people respond well to Arnica and others will require Rhus toxicodendron Ruta graviolens Bryonia and a variety of other cures that are identified by various signs of excessive exertion. There's nothing to say the case that Arnica isn't effective, but it's just that Arnica does not work for patients who require an alternative remedy at the time. Another thing to note is that even for those who require Arnica there are some who might be preferring a 30X or 12C or another dosage. There are far too many aspects that affect homeopathic treatment for an RCT standard to be able to cover all of them.

To make it more adaptable to the RCT method to homeopathy, we have to take their individual character into account. Instead of providing the same medication to all of the patients We'll need to offer every person the appropriate solution for their particular ailments. It's likely that we'll end with a few dozen or more medications for a group that is active of 15 or 20 people. This isn't just a way to defeat the idea of studying the individual medicine one at a but it's also longer-lasting than an RCT. The information needed to pick the right homeopathic treatment can't be collected by mechanical means and requires an eye for detail and a nuanced evaluation performed by an experienced and trained human brain. Every participant participating in clinical trials has to undergo a thorough interview with an experienced homeopath. This could take anywhere from a few to hours. Of course, both the active as well as the participants in the control group must be conducted in the same manner. After that, the homeopaths of the profession are required to study the ailments of each participant in order and determine a specific treatment for each participant, a procedure which can last for several days or hours. This is in violation of one of the primary purposes of RCT design. Its goal is to remove the variability of human judgement as far as is possible. This also means that it is costlier than conventional RCT due to the huge quantity of expert labor required.

It is a major obstacle to funding when it comes to research on homeopathy. Traditional drug trials are funded by pharmaceutical firms, who have the ability to keep a patent for long enough to pay for the substantial expenses of developing and researching. The homeopathic medicines are made of organic substances using a method that has been utilized since the beginning of time therefore there's no chance to patent the homeopathic remedies. This means that the margins for profit for homeopathic companies are lower than the regular ones. The money they receive to conduct research is used for the creation of innovative products for their customers, not conducting studies to confirm that what they have already established that is accurate.

When evaluating clinical trials, it's important to keep in mind the exact question originally asked before the trial was planned at the beginning. Many people view trial trials using homeopathy, and conclude that the issue is "Does homeopathy work?" In reality, the Boston Marathon trial wasn't designed to answer that question. It's not possible to find in a conventional RCT. In addition, no one will conduct a traditional drug study to find out, "Does conventional medicine work?" It is essential to remain sane when we evaluate the results and when designing studies.

The most accurate method to know if homeopathy actually works is to look at the evidence from clinical studies. Homeopaths and other therapists keep meticulous records throughout decades, and they have an abundance of information on its efficacy in every possibility of context. But in conventional medical research, this kind of information is regarded as biased and based on anecdotes. In spite of the volume, evidence isn't sufficient by current methodologies for research.

It's a bit ironic that homeopathy has been accused as not scientifically sound. The people who make the claim often are based on faulty or inaccurate data, and ignore the scientific rigor of homeopathy as well as the mountain of scientifically-based clinical experiences accumulated through the years, which is a naive move. Research that is truly scientific uses instruments and methodologies that match the topic under study and poses questions that research will be able to be able to. Being able to judge homeopathy objectively and fairly requires a thorough understanding of the subject to research it in the right manners - such as placing bananas into banana boxes, and eggs inside egg cartons.

Laboratory Science

For research in the laboratory We're waiting on technologies that can reveal how homeopathy functions. As with many traditional medicines that are used, homeopathy is based upon the notion that it is effective before we know why. We're now beginning to see encouraging results from labs using extremely sensitive instruments, however we have much to be done.

The problem is this. Because they're produced through the process of serial diluting (Chapter 3) Most homeopathic treatments don't contain any from the compounds they're made out of. When you examine them in a laboratory of chemistry, they'll look similar to water. That's probably the main reason why people dismiss the practice of homeopathy and never try to understand it. According to the way used to define medications in the present, "there's nothing in them."

There's actually something extremely powerful about these substances - but it's not what we're used looking for in medicine, or those that we've created tools for.

It's not unexpected to find that "there's nothing in them" argument is convincing. In the way that modern Western medical science (using "medicine" here to refer to treatments different from surgery) has evolved over time, it's almost all of its eggs into the chemistry basket to say. What I am referring to is that since more than 100 years ago research into biochemical processes within living organisms have influenced in the direction of medical research. Medical science has focused its research predominantly on the biological and chemical components of living creatures.

The result of this focus is how we view medical treatment today. Medicines are formulas which we add to our bodies for digestion and eliminated. They are taken in a prescribed order based on the rate at which they're processed. The body's weight is used in calculating doses by anticipating how much medicine our bodies can absorb and then excrete. A dose that is overdosed means that we consumed too much of the drug that our body could not take it in. These practices happen as a result of the fact that medicines contain chemicals and target the chemical processes that occur in our body. In the meantime, we've developed laboratory technologies that are compatible with this method of medicine. As a result, we have more and more information on living organisms' chemistry both in disease and health and further developing chemicals in medicine, and increasing the importance of chemical chemistry. What we ask for determines the responses we receive and, in turn, determine the method we follow.

It's not the only means to impact the health. In the case of conventional medicine, which focuses on chemical processes, homeopathy is a realm of physical science. Living bodies are physical - something we be able to touch and feel and feel, which is the domain of surgery. It's chemical, which is based through biochemical processes, which is which is the domain of chemical medicine as well as electromagnetic, which falls within an area of physics as are energies such as homeopathy. The electromagnetic properties of living beings aren't examined as thoroughly as physical and chemical ones, yet they're just as true. Based on our personal life experience as a the human body that we could be both physical and chemical however, that's not all we're.

According to the most recent research conducted in labs can discern the present that homeopathy operates on an electromagnetism level to trigger changes on both the physical and chemical level. If the potentized remedy is in contact with the electromagnetic aspects of living things and causes an change in energy that reorients the biological process away from disease towards healthy. This phenomenon has been seen repeatedly in the field however it has not yet been studied in depth in the laboratory.

One of the most intriguing laboratory investigations to understand how homeopathy functions is conducted in physics laboratories equipped with instruments that are sensitive enough to recognize the behaviour of nanoparticles that have been found with high-potency homeopathic remedies. The potentized mercury, quinine daisies and bushmaster venom might all appear similar to water when you conduct a chemical analysis However, when you employ modern tools for physics, they're different and each possessing its own distinct magnetic signal.

Nanoparticles can range between one and 100 nanometers in diameter.

They're about as small than soccer balls.

A soccer ball, for example, is much smaller than earth.

There is evidence that suggests that powerful medicines' potency is not due to the diluting process but rather through the agitation employed during their production (Chapter 3.). The medicines that are diluted however not succussed show the same activity as the ones created using the standard method of potentization. Saying that homeopathic drugs are very dilute is not more than half of the truth. Diluted medicines are safe however succussion is what makes them efficient.

The research technology used to study potentized remedies is still in the early stages as compared to the potential it holds, and in the coming decades, we will likely see advancements in laboratory capabilities which could be able to explain the reason for the success that homeopathy has been clinically confirmed to be. What science has to say about homeopathy is Keep an eye out.

Chapter 5: Philosophy

If you look at it, all methods have an underlying philosophy. Any action we make was derived from an concept. It's not often that the concept is explicitly stated, however it's present and influences what we undertake. Understanding the thinking patterns which drive our decisions will help us remain in the right direction and be consistent, making the actions we take efficient. The more conscious we become of the concepts and ideas of what we are doing and the more able us to adhere to the goals we set for ourselves and to improve, change, and develop.

The way we take take care of our bodies is determined by the way we perceive. Are we thinking of our body as an instrument? Then we put our attention on the physics of its operation in terms of its structure and function. Do we view the body to be a flexible, dynamic system? And then we take care of the body by enabling it to react to change in a healthy manner. What about illnesses Do we see it as a threat to an otherwise healthy body, and thus attempt to defeat an enemy that is invading? Do we view the illness as an issue with the human body and seek to address the problem inside?

Naturally, there are many possibilities for any of the above issues, and in the real daily life, we're thinking in several ways simultaneously. Living organisms are physical substance, chemical structure and many more. Things that are not living are also chemical and material However, in contrast to them the living thing includes an electromagnet system that coordinates and animating both the chemical and the material that makes a difference between living things and what you would consider as "life." And then there are the life-like aspects that are metaphysical to living human beings and the components that are referred to as soul, spirits, personalities, other such things. The way we think about this complicated creature will determine how we think about it during healthy and sick conditions and the way we care for it.

In the process of watching again and repeatedly how remedies that are homeopathic work Homeopaths have a better understanding of living creatures and how they can heal. The concept we refer to as "homeopathic philosophy" is not created concepts, but the principles that are derived from observation in clinical settings. These aren't ancient beliefs or knowledge; they're based on experience and are guidelines which we can follow to achieve that we get the results we wish to achieve.

They are applicable for any situation in which we make use of homeopathy. They're useful to homeopathic prescribers and professional practitioners alike. It's the best place to go in the event of an illness we've never encountered previously, as they direct us towards a strategy that is consistent, even if you're not in a familiar areas. They're basically the maps that we use regardless of which direction we travel. They help us decide not only on the way we treat illnesses, as well as how we research the effectiveness of medicines as well as how we evaluate the results. Every good practice in homeopathy is built on solid homeopathic principles. Actually, I'll go as far to claim that you cannot make use of homeopathy in a way that is effective without this.

Vitalist Thinking

The core of homeopathic thought is a method of thinking that is referred to as"vitalism.. It is based on the idea that living creatures are fueled by an inner energy which is the driving force behind their lives. The internal energy that drives them creates the distinction between living things and nonliving ones in spite of how much chemical structure or chemistry they have in common. Vitalism believes that this energy within as the underlying cause of everything that happens within living organisms.

It is easier to comprehend the concept of vitalism when compared to the opposite way of thinking that we are more comfortable with, a concept we call materialism. In this instance, I'm using materialism is not in the sense of wanting to possess lots of things, however, but as a philosophical concept. A philosophy of thought it is a method of thinking which trace the origins of phenomena to the material (physical or structural) chemical) factors.

If, for instance, someone suffers from a sore throat and has a positive test for strep The materialist argument could suggest that bacteria are present in the throat. Bacteria are present even though they're microscopically. The vitalist theory would recognize the presence of bacteria, yet highlight the vulnerability which allowed them to cause problems initially. According to the vitalist view, the most fundamental reason behind the sore throat is because the body wasn't able to fight the bacterial disease. The vulnerability was present before the bacterium was present.

Both of these models contribute to different research methods. For instance, in the case of strep-throph where the emphasis is on pathogens the more we know about them, the more we will be able to eradicate them, or even stop the spread of infection to people. It is important to understand how they are living and where they originate from the factors that strengthen and weaken their ability to fight, and so on. However an emphasis on the susceptibility and resilience of a person's body will lead to studies on how to maintain health as well as what our body is doing when it is ill.

The two concepts of materialism and vitalism can result in different strategies for treatment. If the cause of sore throat is due to bacteria, it's obvious it is best to eliminate the bacteria, and take whatever steps are necessary to stop exposure to it again. When the bacteria have gone and eliminated, it's expected that the end result is the return of good health. A clean strep test after treatment confirms success. If the issue stems from what's going on within the throat, expert care is the most effective option. Experts in whatever area of the body has symptoms is the one most qualified to treat it. In contrast when the reason is an organism's vulnerability to infection, treating the issue on a deeper and larger scale is the better option than eliminating the bacteria. When the organism gets more robust, bacteria won't become a concern for it anymore. A vitalist perspective results in a holistic approach since susceptibility runs through the entire organism regardless of the location where infection might appear currently. The proof that therapy has been successful is not just from the disappearance of infections, but also from the better functioning of the human body in general.

In this particular explanation I've created a simplified explanation in order to draw out the distinctions between these two methods of thinking. There is no one who believes in only one either way - this could be absurd because living things are both animating and material. And each aspect of these must be considered. The majority of health-related practices incorporate both vitalist and materialist thought however the focus differs from one belief system to the next. The current medical system is based on the materialist perspective, while homeopathy is a vitalist perspective.

There is evidence of vitalism that is present in homeopathy through the types of remedies that we take: the energetic that are not physical ones. This is also the reason for homeopathy's thorough procedure of taking cases, which is to discover all ways that the vital force manifesting its state above the issue. This is the basis for our evaluation of remedies' actions: if issues are treated from the inside it is a planned approach for how the process will progress. Vitalism is a major factor in the goal of our work that isn't just to eliminate symptoms, but also in order to restore the body into its highest state of well-being.

The Vital Force

Homeopaths refer to the energy within that animates a living thing the vital force. It's the same as the concept that Traditional Chinese Medicine calls chi. Vital force is a physical force, similar to gravity or magnetism. As with magnetism and gravity however, it cannot be felt by touching or sight, hear, and other senses. But it can be observed by its results. Similar to all natural forces, it acts in regular, predictable manners. If we are interested in knowing what it is doing, we could see it within living organisms And with the proper tools, we could study the physics of it within labs as well.

Each living organism is unique and is a unique organism with its own force. Certain properties are universally which are common to all living things but also some specific to every. Your vital force is what drives, organizes, and controls every activity within your body. It decides how your digestion operates, what health issues you're susceptible to, the way your immune system reacts to illness, and even the way you process your thoughts and emotional responses - basically each and every function you perform. Your vital energy with your mind or intention the way you control gravity or magnetic force.

Though the power of vitality is not material, it's not religious or spiritual. It doesn't have any religious significance and there's a broad range of religions among homeopaths from all over the world. Hahnemann identified the vital force as "spirit-like," but he utilized the term "spirit" in the sense of "ghost," not in the sense of "spiritual." In his writings, Hahnemann refers to both the soul as well as the vital force. He clarifies that they are two distinct entities. Philosophies and religions disagree regarding the question about whether or not the soul is real as a thing, how it functions and what it is what it does in its behavior, etc. In contrast, the essential power is the natural phenomenon. The question of whether or not something is an soul can be subject to interpretation. However, whether it's alive, is simply an unavoidable truth.

Vital force is flexible and creative. Being a force for creativity, it's at the heart of all organism's structure and actions. It's why living things develop. It controls all of our daily actions, including making the energy we need from food, creating thoughts and ideas, and controlling all the biochemical process which keeps us alive. Being a receptive force, it responds to events and stimulation that come from the outside. It's the motor for our immune system's response to harmful bacteria and viruses as well as our swelling and bruises in the aftermath of injuries, the pain warning us of risk, the processing of the information that the senses provide as well as our emotional reactions such as the emotion of grief or anger to the events of our lives. All that living creatures can do, but nonliving organisms don't are a result of this vital power of the force.

Health and Illness

If your body is in good health, everything functions well. You're feeling good and are in control of what's right for your needs. If your vital power is compromised, it can cause the same problems that are specific for your situation. The consequences that occur when the vital force is affected will be unique to the individual the same way as how it works when it's in tune. Every person has their individual areas of vulnerability as well as our own personal habits. When we're healthy or sick our bodies are always energized by the force of life and are always our individual selves.

The words we employ to talk about the force behind it is symbolic. It's difficult to assign concrete words on ineffable objects. Hahnemann stated the vital force as possibly "mistuned," which keeps the vital force from functioning properly. Others who translate the text choose "deranged," "untuned," or "disturbed" to convert Hahnemann's original German to English. Homeopaths also make use of words such as "impaired," "blocked," "struggling," "misdirected," "hindered," "weakened," and so on.

What is it that makes one's vital force to work more effectively or less effectively? There are many variables however they're not always the way you'd think. Lifestyle and diet, thinking about and goals, physical exercise and rest don't "derange" the vital force. They are extremely beneficial by helping or deter the vital force to keep the body in good condition however they do not influence its basic condition. Like you could fold a paper plane to assist or thwart gravity, you are able to consume food, drink or sleep with ways that can either aid or derail the vital force. The way you fold the airplane isn't a factor in determining gravity. And the way you eat or drink, rest, and conduct your life doesn't alter the force of your life.

The causes which "mistune" the vital force can be more complex. Certain health-related tendencies that we have inherited from our past ancestors have been encoded in our vital energy right from the beginning and not necessarily in genetics but rather in the language of vital energy. As a result, the majority of people of today suffer from some degree or "mistunement." Sustained suppression of its symptoms could cause a mistuning of the vital force. Certain ailments and types of trauma may affect the vital force, making it in a position to not return your body back to its previous condition of wellness.

If our vital force is disoriented, it can cause problems with any or all aspects of our daily functioning. This vital force is the same one that drives all of us. As such, it's effects from mistuning could manifest in any part of the human body, and within any field or multiple one. As an example, you could struggle to combat viruses or healing from injuries or even begin the course of developing a chronic condition or be struggling with self-defeating thought patterns and thoughts. It is possible that you are fatigued, having trouble sleeping with nightmares or other behavior issues, experience menstrual cramps and migraines, or urinary infections, and develop the appearance of cysts, atrophy, or other pathological growths, or any of a variety of different possibilities. If the symptoms are intermittent instead of constant you may notice that the mistunedness in your vital power is present all the time even if you're feeling well.

We can rid the vital force from its misalignment using homeopathy. The language of the vital force is not chemistry but energy therefore it requires the energy medicine in order to rectify the imbalance. Similar to lifestyle and diet choices chemicals can aid or hinder for the vital force perform however they aren't able to improve its basic condition. Homeopathy's powerful medicines communicate in the language spoken by Vital Force.

A solution at the level of the vital force will result in better functioning all over. The vital force gets more robust and thus will withstand higher stress levels without causing signs. The body is able to fight acute conditions quickly and with no permanent repercussions. It also reverses the development of chronic illness signs and symptoms. It improves the ability to perceive precisely and reacting appropriately to mental, physical and emotional triggers we come across. This can lead to the feeling of happiness that permeates all areas of our life.

Chapter 6: How to Start

If you're looking to give the traditional homeopathic method a go it's possible to follow the footsteps of thousands across the globe who've benefitted of this incredible treatment. Patients of medical professionals, customers of homeopaths who are professionals, students at study groups and schools and even home prescribers for their families. There's plenty of information as well as a wealth of sources available to help you. No matter what your goals and needs the homeopathic approach will aid you in reaching them.

There are two basic locations where homeopathy can be found within the U.S. today: at the home or with the assistance of a licensed practitioner. There are some hospitals that offer homeopathic treatment elsewhere, but they are not available in the United States. It is used at home by any person who wishes to assist their family members who suffers from minor illnesses and is keen to understand some basic concepts. When it comes to professional settings, it's the responsibility of specialists who can assist to solve more difficult and complex problems. Every setting has various purposes. You'll need to evaluate your requirements and objectives to determine what to do first. Whichever option you pick, or the other, you're sure to experience a change in your life positively in stunning ways.

The practice of homeopathy is constant throughout all environments and has been that way since its inception. Innovative approaches, innovative technologies, and even discoveries of the writings of Hahnemann that were previously undiscovered are helping homeopathy to evolve and the practice remains steady and consistent.

The home care provider as well as professional homeopaths adhere to the exact same procedure. They differ on the scale of what they're examining. For home-based care of injuries or acute conditions, we tend to focus only on a few symptoms and an ephemeral amount of duration. When it comes to professional treatment, the homeopath generally considers all aspects of a person's life over in the past, decades or the entire life span. Meticulous information-gathering, orderly reasoning, careful research, and keen observation are all crucial in both settings. An organized and consistent method is equally important in homeopathy just like it is with conventional medicine or in any other form of treatment.

If you're looking to start your journey at home This method is the guide. There's only something else you'll need to be aware of.

Acute and Chronic. Chronic

The first step is to must be able to distinguish an acute condition from one that is chronic. It is crucial as you may take care of acute ailments yourself, however you must seek out a specialist for chronic diseases. The idea of treating an ongoing ailment like it's acute is among the most frequent mistakes made by home-based prescribers however, distinguishing them from each other is more difficult than it appear.

Let's look at my son who's story can be found part II of the book. There were ear infections, and streptococcal infections. Each time, a new infection would come and go but in the midst of them his body was feeling great and went about the world with enthusiasm.

In one sense it was that he was a health young man with occasional acute illness. Each illness had its own event with a distinct start and an end. This is a part of the definition of an illness that is acute which is confined to a limited duration, frequently with an abrupt start that was the same style. Every child, excluding the very few who do not get sick, is afflicted with acute illness every now and then. My son was healthy and normal kid.

Homeopaths have discovered in the past that chronic illnesses that repeat similar to one another can be a sign of chronic illness and are more difficult to manage. It's not an individual incident but the susceptibility which causes them to repeat themselves. Like we saw when my son was sick eliminating each illness in the short-term did not solve the issue over the long term. The issue didn't matter if we tried an antibiotic or a natural treatment specifically targeting the issue The infections continued to come. Then, when he received constitutional therapy with a professional traditional homeopath.

What do you need to know when you're in need of a medical professional? One good rule to follow is to ensure that you looked to a doctor prior to learning about homeopathy, it's time to consult an expert. It's not just for emergencies obviously. If this is an incident that's isolated that you've walked to a pharmacy to help it be treated at home, then it's suitable to test your own homeopathic prescription skills for a test. A good rule of thumb is should something appear to be urgent condition but isn't resolved by the best home remedies then it might be a chronic illness.

When you've mastered the art of distinguishing the difference between chronic and acute, it's time to be confidently transition towards home-based treatment.

Home Care

If you want to begin using remedies at home with homeopathy All you require is some books and an aid kit, or perhaps a local store with remedies for homeopathy.

The first thing I tried was an assortment of remedies for thirty-six of a top homeopathic company. The cost was less than hundred dollars, and was packaged with a durable, sturdy plastic container. Kits can be a great option to get started with your DIY collection of remedies as the price per treatment is usually lower than purchasing the remedies individually. The options are endless: each manufacturer has a variety of remedies included in their kits. And in the end, you'll likely require specific remedies that are available in a range of different potencies. My initial kit was the 30C version, but the 30X and 12C kits are equally effective. Soon I had augmented my supplies with different solutions that were necessary in my circles. It is a good idea to build on the kits you begin with.

There are databases and apps designed to analyse the symptoms you type in and give the name of the treatment to recommend. Be wary of these apps and databases. However well-studied they may be and the famed homeopaths that wrote them are, they're not able to reproduce the multi-dimensional thinking required to select a remedy. It is a bit more beneficial to use websites offering an index of searchable medical conditions, as well as a narrowed options of treatment options to choose from. However, here too the writers (this is me, too) have removed many of the details in order to keep it short. Whichever reference tool which you select, you need to be proficient in the process of analyzing a case, and know the right information to incorporate into the analysis process, and these is something that software cannot take care of for you.

The fact is that a brain that is well-equipped and equipped is the most effective prescriber. The majority of home health books will explain the steps to analyze a situation and determine what's crucial in selecting a treatment after which with some repetition, you'll soon be able to do it. After you've completed the case and identified which signs are the most crucial for your treatment plan You'll then compare the remedies and find the one that best suits the most important aspects of the case. In order to be completely prepared, you need many sources for information. Electronic sources can be one of your options, but you'll find so many excellent guides on this subject and you'd be foolish not to get a copy.

Many books and databases geared towards the home-based prescriber are divided into diseases and, under each, they provide brief profiles of the ailments that are suitable for the remedy. As an example, if you browse through the section on coughs, you might find the dry cough which is difficult and more severe at night requires this treatment, or a cough worse after eating but better by a cooler breeze, calls for another remedy. This may seem straightforward, however when I was an RN, there was no one that could be matched precisely. It's due to the fact that there are numerous ways in which an illness can manifest itself for different individuals. It is essential to have enough knowledge to be able to make an informed choice of what the treatment your symptoms require and not in a way that it overpowers the patient. When I was a doctor in acute need of prescriptions I was carrying eight to 10 home health books, and would choose whichever two or three offered the most concise and the most comprehensive information on the condition I was doing research on at the moment.

The home health books provide recommendations on dosage, potency, frequency as well as the length of time you should be patient for the remedy to take effect before attempting an alternative. A few of them provide background information about the subject and also suggestions on how to handle your case. A few provide advice about how to determine the most significant symptoms to address with your treatment. Some of my favorites also tell you the best time to contact a physician or go to emergency treatment.

If you begin practicing homeopathy in your home, it's likely that you'll be hungry to talk with other practitioners at home. The practice of homeopathy is still a rarity in many areas, which is why social media is a good option to help. There are some regions that have group study sessions in person that include guests speakers library lending, particular events, and many more. A membership at a low cost to the National Center for Homeopathy grants access to a variety of online educational materials as well as printed in books, discounted tickets to their national conferences, and much more. If you'd like to gain knowledge from experienced instructors Some of the institutions who train professional homeopaths provide homeopathic courses in person or on the web. Just like everything else, make sure you verify the authenticity of the provider you're relying on to ensure precise information.

The one drawback to being a doctor at home is similar as owning an automobile: everybody is likely to need your assistance. That's not necessarily a bad issue, as each when you examine a patient and suggest a treatment it's a chance to learn and also aiding. This also provides you with a an opportunity to teach other people on homeopathy and witness the enthusiasm of others grow along as does yours.

Since I began using homeopathy in my the home level, I experienced a condition which I've learned to recognize to be a problem for new prescribers The reason I was adamant about giving every patient a remedy. Every bruise or bump and every bug bite or any sting or tear, and every sorrow following losing a beloved pet every situation seemed to require intervention using these seemingly magic white crystals. When I saw a small incident or read a tale and then think "I know the remedy for that!" If the same thing happens to you be reminded of the natural wisdom. It's not always necessary to help as living things are self-healing and should be given the opportunity to perform first. Being a holistic practitioner, either at the home or in a professional situation, doesn't mean providing cures. It's about helping nature whenever it's in need of help as well as standing by in the event that you don't.

Professional Care

However, even if you are a highly skilled homeopathic practitioner it is likely to certain things to be being left to experts. If you are a trained experienced practitioner, homeopathy can transform your life. The most skilled practitioners of classical homeopathy have completed intense training for a number of several years, and have successfully passed the gruelling examinations, and proved their expertise through rigorous practical training. They use a lot of the same treatments that are available on the counter for use for yourself, the professionals understand each disease and medication deeper, and are competent to direct the force of nature towards the highest level of wellness. Classical homeopathy has reached its Gold Standard when it's under the care of trained professionals.

The type of work professional homeopaths are often described in the context of "constitutional care." This is a flimsy word because it's got distinct meanings in various instances. Homeopathy is typically applied to refer to professional treatment that addresses all aspects of the individual. However, it doesn't mean that they believe that people fall into the categories of constitutionality, as does for instance, Ayurveda or Tibetan medicine. The way we think about each patient is as an person. However, this doesn't mean that professionals at homeopaths try to identify your primary character, as we understand the fact that living organisms evolve over the course of. The practice of homeopathy is called constitutional care. is a method that provides an all-encompassing view of the patient, including the entirety of who they are both in the present and over their lifetime. The most common use of it is for chronic illnesses.

The majority of professional homeopaths are not specialists. They don't treat specific ailments but rather, we're trying to help the vital force's efforts to improve the health of people. Vital force is the exact natural force that exists in everyone from all races, ages or gender identities, religions etc. As we gain experience in dealing with all kinds of illnesses in different types of individuals more prepared us to recognize and address each and every new and individual vital force that comes to our attention. Our practice is largely a generalist and treat every case as a whole.

Regarding their history However, there exist a myriad of traditional homeopaths. They include medical professionals like nurses, doctors, practitioners, naturopathic doctors veterinarians, acupuncturists as well as others. Some of them use only homeopathy, while others utilize it alongside other methods. Additionally, there are professional homeopaths in the non-medical community who specialize in homeopathy. What kind of homeopath best suits your needs is based on your personal preferences as well as their accessibility in your region.

The two types of homeopaths may decide to pursue the certification of homeopathy. The medical certificate doesn't necessarily indicate that someone is a professional in homeopathy. To ensure a homeopath's ability, verify their certifications in homeopathy. The section on Resources in the final section of this publication contains several reliable, independent organizations for certifying. For instance, the Council for Homeopathic Certification (CHC) is one of the largest with the highest quality standards for their certification procedure which is accessible to physicians and non-medical professionals that satisfy the educational requirements. For CHC certification, non-medical practitioners need to have sufficient experience in medical treatment to know those who are in medical danger or requires an appointment with a conventional practitioner, to ensure you are assured that you are in good hands. CHC certification requires a specific lengthy training course, along with the supervision of the clinical practitioner, as well as a series of tests. To keep their certifications for both medical and non-medical homeopaths must abide by an uncompromising code of ethics as well as meet regular professional requirements for development. The certification specifically for homeopathy can be a sign that a homeopath is licensed.

The best option is to choose the person with the highest experience in homeopathy available. In terms of getting outcomes, medical and non-medical homeopaths can be alike. There is no difference in whether they've treated the condition you're experiencing before and will be searching to find the treatment that matches you, not the condition you're suffering from. The homeopath will be entrusting you to handle not just the health of your body but also with lots of information about you and so it's important that you are at ease with the person. Many homeopaths will chat with them on the phone for about a minute for no cost so that they can meet the other person before making an appointment. A few are even willing to offer the opportunity to meet with them in person, for no cost.

Professionals may practice via remote conference to improve their reach because a lot of areas in the nation are not served. A lot of people do not prefer to do it because they are dependent upon the type of observations that is only possible in person. Others have begun to develop remote case-taking as a particular capability. Another aspect to consider when taking into consideration your desires and requirements. A lot of people don't have to visit their homeopath as frequently, therefore traveling a distance is normal.

If you go to an expert homeopath for the first time, your initial consultation could last 90 minutes or longer. The homeopath may ask you to complete a lengthy background form prior to arriving but they'll still be asking you a variety of questions pertaining to every part of your daily life. They'll ask about areas of your life that appear not to have anything to do with your reason for being there However, as the constitutional treatment you receive will cover every one parts of you, this matters. The doctor will likely inquire what your primary concerns are thoroughly, as well as gather data about your overall health such as your interests and preferences along with your personality and many more. A man I spoke to after the first visit "Now you know me better than anyone else on earth - including my wife." This degree of specificity will allow your homeopath to determine which remedy most closely matches your needs. With more than three thousand treatments available, many that look alike, it's not an easy process to determine the most appropriate one.

The benefits of homeopathy are particularly beneficial for youngsters, who's vital force can be very sensitive. The method of interviewing is tailored to the child's stage of development. My typical approach to youngsters is to provide the children some art or toys tools and watch how they engage in play, while asking questions to their parents. I will also allow the parents an hour to be with me since there might be concerns or stories that should not be shared before the child. The child isn't doing anyone any harm to listen to their parents talk to strangers about their thoughts on what they think is "wrong" with them. Teens usually can be able to handle similar conversations as adults when their parents are waiting out in the cold, however sensitivity the level of comfortability of a person is crucial regardless of the age.

After the initial consultation, the homeopath could take some time to research what you've provided them prior to being certain about which treatment to suggest. It's not uncommon for me to make a final decision just after several weeks or even more the massive collection of books accessible to professional. In addition to their recommendation for a remedy the homeopath can provide you with instructions about how to use the remedy, and possibly on ways to increase its efficacy. The majority of them will ask for you to not take any alternative to the one they prescribe, therefore it is important to keep the attention of your homeopath on other ailments.

The best approach to constitutional care is using a longer-term approach. A lot of homeopaths set the first appointment to follow up longer than six weeks after the treatment is completed to ensure that it's got enough time to work. In general, ailments that develop over time, which is what most chronic diseases do, can require time to heal. If you're experiencing some urgent or urgent issue it is likely that a quicker examination may be necessary. Your homeopath might not know when your remedy will take effect or for how long you'll require treatments. The vitality of your body is the primary judge of your own speed of healing. Homeopathy does not aim for rapid results but rather slow and steady improvement over time.

The majority of health insurance policies cover the homeopathic treatment only when your homeopath is certified medically, it's very cost-effective due to its beneficial effects on general well-being. My family of four began to pay out of pocket for an acupuncturist, our overall cost of health insurance decreased since we were paying lower copays. Because homeopathic remedies cost so little they are primarily on the part of the practitioner's time. Professional homeopaths typically bill their services in a manner comparable to Therapists, although you'll meet your homeopath less frequently as an Therapist. The main expense will be when you begin the treatment since follow-up appointments typically are smaller than your initial appointment.

Practitioners should not claim to deliver outcomes. They should charge reasonable fees and comparable to other practitioners within the field, and they must explain their charges and policies on payment upfront. They should behave courteously and courteous and be able to respond to your inquiries clearly. They must adhere to the same rules regarding confidentiality that the therapist would and should be willing to discuss the ethics of their practice upon your the request of. Every time you interact with them you must feel like you're working with an expert.

The accounts that are in the second part of the book provide an overview of the variety of illnesses I've helped treat by homeopathy. However, be aware that homeopathy is not the same as magic. It can take several unsuccessful attempts before you find the perfect solution. Particularly if you've tried other remedies or have an ongoing condition It could take a few several weeks or even months before you notice changes. The homeopathic remedies have a distinct course of action than standard medicines and they are effective even after you've taken the pills, and there could occur ups and downs during their effects. The best way to get the most value for your money is to make use in time and money when you follow up with the treatment your doctor recommends, and providing her with minimum six to nine months for results before thinking about switching your homeopath. However, even if you're certain your remedy is working or not performed, make sure you the next visit because your homeopath might offer a different viewpoint which will help you move forward. They could be able determine, long before indicators are apparent for you, that your treatment will yield what you expect as well as how to adjust your regimen to improve the effectiveness of it. Your doctor is the only one who can truly understand the whole story, and they'll be the first to determine what's going on. Routinely checking in even when doing well will help maintain your progress and may even help you steer back future troubles.

One of the great benefits of constitutional medicine at home is the depth of its coverage. You can't count how many times you've sought assistance to treat a particular ailment, but then found that the rest are also cured. Things that you've gotten used to living with, that it's hard to notice these issues can go away and allow you to be more relaxed than you might. A woman I spoke to said "After the remedy I lost my taste for alcohol, and looking back, I see that I had a drinking problem even though I was denying it." The woman sought help in a different area and hadn't mentioned any alcohol consumption at the time of our first meeting, however, her life force changed and led her towards a new way of life that was more beneficial for her. As time passed, her concerns caused her to seek the homeopathic treatment were also resolved.

The benefits of homeopathy are a great alternative to a healthcare plan that incorporates various other approaches, such as traditional medical practices. The homeopath can advise you regarding how homeopathy could fit within your overall healthcare. When you have an entire team set up it will be easier to make educated choices that will help you maintain your overall health despite the difficulties life throws at you.

Chapter 7: What is Health

It is that great feeling of feeling free and liberated from the pressures and stress that come with daily life. It is the ability to pursue your desires, achieve your goals, and enjoy fully. Being able to realize your goals and feel confident. There are strains and stressors for everyone within their lives. Health does not mean being free of them but rather living your life free of being burdened due to them.

Happiness and happiness are the foundation of health. Being content in your body and mind. The ability to quickly adjust and overcome any difficulties you encounter.

The concept of health could vary from person to person. What are the best way to determine the health of your body? It's a great idea to think about the meaning of health to you.

What are your health-related goals?

What are you looking to see improved?

Are you covered under longer-term health plan?

How do you want to oversee your family's health care?

Do you consider yourself healthy?

If you suffer from recurring or chronic illnesses Are you living your life as you would like to?

Are your children healthy?

It is my opinion the concept of health as physical, emotional or mental. To me, peace of mind and satisfaction is essential. Therefore, if you are suffering from specific health concerns but you are still enjoying a healthy and happy existence.

What is Ill Health

Health problems are a result of a lack of peace, contentment and inner peace.

Health problems can cause mental, physical or emotional symptoms that aren't able to be resolved. Stress, depression, anxiety or sadness. Traumas from the past that have detrimental effects on your lifestyle and capacity to deal with it.

Being held back or stifled in a manner, but with no feeling of peace, or happiness. Becoming weighed down with the strains and stresses that are part of daily life.

Are there any people on this world who's healthy and happy? I doubt it! We are all striving to be the best we could be.

What is Homeopathy

The homeopathic method is a holistic alternative to conventional medicine. The basic premise of homeopathy is that it 'like cures like'

Homeopathic remedies are created by combining the mineral, plant as well as animal kingdoms. Similar to energetic blueprints of their physical forms (eg. the energy blueprint of the actual bee). The effects a chemical can cause in its physical structure and can be treated with its homeopathic counterpart (eg. Apis from bees, is used to treat bites or stings Allium Cepa composed of the red onion and is a remedy for Hayfever). They function as a catalyst that stimulates the Vital Force (your energy self). However, the signs of a person must be in line with the symptoms that the remedy is aiming to treat. It is crucial, or the cure will not work.

Many homeopathic remedies are readily available. However, the majority of people who use at-home homeopathy for treating their families and friends will opt for the best Acute remedies (approx. 40-50) that are described by this publication.

Professional homeopaths are known to use alternative methods and I think that the majority of homeopaths remain within 200 treatments all through their careers.

The holistic method of homeopathy provides a comprehensive method of health that treats individuals as a whole instead of focusing on the disease label. The symptoms on every level are to be considered when deciding on the best remedy that matches that addresses the emotional and mental aspects of physical.

It is possible to use homeopathy alongside traditional medicines - the decision is yours

Benefits of Homeopathy

Safe & gentle

Non-toxic

Non-addictive

It is easy to manage, especially infants and children

Safe during pregnancy

OK to utilize in conjunction with other treatments, medications or therapies

All ages are safe and all stages of life

Soft yet strong

Provides an all-encompassing solution of people who are interested in an approach to natural health

It is easily accessible - via online pharmacies that specialize in homeopathy and health food shops

Empowering

Acute -v- Chronic Illness

This book is geared towards aiding you in treating acute illnesses at your home. The term "acute illness" refers to a quick, self-limiting ailment that should resolve its own way, if given enough the time. It's not a chronic condition and is unlikely to have lasting negative effects. There are many homeopathic treatments that can be used to treat acute illnesses.

The chronic illness gets more severe that develops with time, and sufferers will notice an increase in their wellbeing and health. The body is in equilibrium, and it seeks out assistance. Homeopathic treatments can be prescribed for chronic illnesses, however it is recommended take advice from the homeopath.

In the case of recurring complaints, specifically for children, may be managed quickly in an incident. It is however a great suggestion to visit an experienced homeopath, who can take an approach that addresses the predisposition as well as susceptibility to the frequent complaint.

Home prescribing may require additional guidance from a homeopath, especially if the condition persists without a cure reaction. Another remedy or potency could be required.

If you are prescribing at home for acute illnesses, it is important to should only treat the symptoms that are associated with the specific acute condition. Other ongoing or persistent symptoms are not considered part of the acute illness and ought to be dealt with in a separate manner.

What is a Constitutional Remedy

The constitutional solution is an amalgamation of nature and nurture

You were made to be

What's happened in your life?

What traits from your genetic heritage could you have been born with?

Which ailments and conditions have a predisposition to

Your temperament and character traits

The use of constitutional treatment is not typically needed when treating chronic complaints. As homeopathy is holistic you can treat a person in the way they are currently in the present, and if it is a chronic problem the symptomology of the issue should be taken into consideration to select the appropriate solution for them at the moment. Find the remedy that matches the symptoms of acute.

The truth is that constitutional intervention isn't always necessary in the case of chronic illness also. Naturally, it's dependent upon the case but it is true that finding the right constitutional solution for a particular person isn't always beneficial. The best approach is to address the patient right at the time and focusing on the symptoms and signs that are displayed as well as the subsequent symptoms. The constitutional layer usually lies under the layer of presenting as are other layers. This is the place where homeopaths and acute prescribers may be lost.

What is an Homeopath do?

The homeopath will examine your or your child's, by taking note of and recording a lot of data about you as well as your characteristic characteristics and signs for example:

Symptoms that are present

A complete history of the patient, including persistent or recurring complaints

What issues need to be dealt with today? (uppermost)

General characteristics

Sleep

Diet

Personality

and many and much more. ....

It is then reviewed and remedies investigated to determine the most appropriate remedy or remedies for the individual. It can be a long and complicated process since most of us live very complicated life and a long history.

The remedies you receive are part of the prescription you receive. Certain homeopaths provide the treatments themselves, while others provide the prescription together with information about the nearest or on-line homeopathic pharmacy. Some homeopaths choose to provide the remedy themselves since the relationship between a doctor, patient and remedies is unique, especially for chronic conditions.

Treatments are generally prescribed over a period of time before a follow-up appointment is needed to evaluate the reaction of the remedy and determine the next actions.

The reaction to remedy is unique and individual. Certain people respond quickly, whereas others have a slower burn. The only way to determine what you're dealing with taking your prescribed treatment and then observe the results.

The majority of homeopaths have an online presence, however not all. Consider asking the area you live in to get recommendations. A few homeopaths are skilled in marketing and business but many do not. Therefore, just because the homeopath doesn't have an social media presence or even bad one, it isn't a reason to conclude that they're not competent in the work they perform. They are generally kind, compassionate, and gentle people so they often are hesitant to share their information online on social media.

If you are considering a homeopath to you, it's an excellent idea to connect with three or four people to begin and then see who you can are able to connect with, and who is to be the best fit for your needs.

Home Prescribing

The term "home prescribing" is that is used to describe the process of selecting treatments for themselves, the children of their family members. This can be done with any assistance from a homeopath and is according to the symptoms that are present. The majority of home-based prescribers possess a collection of remedies at home that they are able to access whenever they require. If the treatment they are looking for does not exist in their store or available, they can buy it on the internet or get it from a family member.

Home prescribing physicians often take small courses in conjunction with homeopaths in order to understand the basic concepts in order to start. After that, they are taught by the experience of others and conduct research based on their individual requirements.

Home-prescribers are typically adept in the use of homeopathy. If you're new to homeopathy, the skills is likely to come to you It just takes some time.

History of Homeopathy

There is a wealth of information available on the web about this subject that I'm not going include the history of the evolution of homeopathy in this work. You can search the internet for blog posts and articles (and books) for additional information about this.

The founder of the company is thought to have been Samuel Hahnemann and I'm providing an overview of his life here.

Samuel Hahnemann

Samuel Hahnemann was born on the 10th of April in 1755 Germany. This was the time that saw political turmoil and change. His family was affluent and his father put a huge importance to the education of his children. He was a highly intelligent and talented young man. He excelled at math, languages, geometry and botany.

He was a chemist and doctor at various institutions while also conducting lectures and translating in order in order to cover the costs. After nine years of practice and chemistry, he began to become frustrated with the standard treatments for cures of the day and decided to stop his work and began to concentrate on studies, research writing and translating.

In this period, Hahnemann translated a book with an essay that explained the reasons why Peruvian Bark, also known as Cinchona (which is now referred to as the remedy for homeopathy China) proved to be effective in treatment of malaria. It also attributed the bitterness the bark of Peru to be the reasons for its effectiveness. Hahnemann was skeptical about this idea and opted to conduct several experiments on his own. He started by taking tiny doses of his own and discovered the symptoms were similar to those of malaria. It was a major factor for the homeopathic process to develop. He carried out further tests on the family members and acquaintances of his and verified his findings that Cinchona had similar symptoms as malaria, a condition is known to treat. This test procedure was known as "proving". It was referred to as similia similibus actualur, meaning. allow like to be cured by similar. This was the very first principle of what he termed homeopathy. The word "homeopathy" was derived by combining the Greek homoios which means the same, as well as pathos that means disease or suffering.

After this, Hahnemann conducted many 'provings in which he observed the signs that any chemical produces when administered to an uninjured person. Hahnemann also examined the symptoms exhibited in the victims of poisonings that were accidental. He then set up a medical practices again, using the data he'd obtained from his research. The methods he used were mocked by doctors, however patients flooded into the clinic and his theories were confirmed by the research results.

Following the demise of Hahnemann in 1843, knowledge of and practice of homeopathy been greatly expanded and extensively in the last century, and we currently are able to access thousands of natural remedies.

Additional information about the history and development of homeopathy may be accessed in full online or in numerous books on homeopathy.

Prescribing Homeopathic Treatment

The homeopathic remedy is chosen through the matching of a patient's symptoms photo with a remedy. Each homeopathic remedy comes with an image that is associated with it. It provides all of the symptoms and symptoms of that particular remedy. Every remedy has strong signs and indicators, which are referred to as the keynotes. These are the symptoms and signs that really stick out and are evident.

In the event of an individual being sick it is normal for them to show indicators and signs of disease. If, for instance, someone suffers from a head cold one of the symptoms could include :

A green vapor from the nostril

pale face

fatigued

thirsty

It's also known as a patient's symptom image. The best remedy for homeopathy is about matching the image of the symptom with the treatment photo.

If you suspect that someone that you take care of is sick, the very first step is to take the instance. Utilize the information gathered from the case-taking process to determine what the most effective treatment for them.

This is how you can do it. ....

Chapter 8: Taking the Case & Deciding on Best Remedy

Note down all of the individual's symptoms, including physical, general, and emotional issues. Be open to questions, but avoid from putting words into their mouth. Keep a note of the things you notice, smell or feel as well as what's happened lately in their lives and what solutions they've tried in the past that worked effectively for them? additional information.

Search for the illness or complaint in the ailments Section within this book.

Find the solution that most closely matches your individual signs and symptoms.

Look up the remedy in the Remedies Section of the book for further clarification and additional information.

The symptoms mentioned for the treatment do not need to exist on the individual. Just try to identify with the symptoms which are the most similar to those in your specific case.

Example Case 1

Child age 5. The child is suffering from a sore throat and has been feeling miserable. There is eczema around their knees and elbows that was first noticed at age one. The eczema is swollen and makes the skin pink underneath. In the evening, the eczema is very itchy. It is possible to get an irritation in their left ear, but in the present, their ears are in good shape. Most symptoms of sore throat include pain when taking liquids or eating food. the throat becomes painful, red and inflamed as you examine it the ear, and there are white spots that appear at the end of the left side of the tonsil. The breath of the patient has that sour scent. They are hot.

Which signs should be considered to treat this acute condition?

The throat is painful

Aches in the throat after swallowing

Throat red

The throat is inflamed

White spots on left tonsil,

Fresh breath smells

A fever or high temperature

Which signs should not be considered in this particular acute condition?

The symptoms that are related to Eczema

A tendency for develop ear infections, as there are no symptoms or signs, currently, this

Ear infections and Eczema are treated separately

Which is the best solution to match?

Find Sore Throats under the section on ailments in the book.

Check out all of the popular solutions and pick the most appropriate one to match your needs.

Make sure you verify this information by checking at the remedy you are looking for in the Remedies section of the book.

You can then administer your selected treatment

What is the best option for me?

Merc-viv (Merc-sol)

Example Case 2

Two years old child. Extremely clingy. This child has always been a clingy child. It seems like she is coming down with something. It started suddenly over the final one hour. Children are thirstier than normal as well as sneezing intermittently. The nose has begun to flow with clear discharge and is streaked in red. The child is suffering from constipation, which began around 6 months of age. Also, they suffered from colic during the initial 4 months of their lives. Mother was able to have a normal pregnancies, however the birth itself of the baby was extremely painful.

What symptoms are appropriate to treat this acute condition?

Sudden onset

Thirsty

Sneezing

Clear, clear discharge, with streaks of red (blood)

What are the symptoms that should not be considered in this particular acute situation?

Clingy, because a child will be generally clingy. If this is a brand new behavior and the child is in acute pain, we should include it.

Constipation is not a part of this more serious condition. It is a separate issue to be addressed.

Colic history and traumatism at birth are not part of this case.

Which is the most suitable solution to match?

Find Colds under the Ailments Section of the book.

Go through the various treatments and choose the most appropriate one to match the symptoms you are experiencing.

Check this information by looking at the remedy you are looking for in the Remedies section of this book.

You can then administer the solution

What is the best option for me?

Phosphorous

If you're looking to pick Aconite due to its sudden beginning, or the Pulsatilla as a result due to the clinginess, which can be fine. I'd suggest Phosphorous due to the blood-stained mucous provides a great emphase to this treatment. Phosphorous is also a lover of company like Pulsatilla (but because of various reasons) However, if Phosphorous is extremely always clingy, then this does not fit into the acute condition.

Administering your Chosen Remedy - General Guideline

Find the solution that best is compatible with your situation.

Start with one tablet. Use the dosage and Frequency instructions in this book.

If an improvement in the response can be received, there is no reason to try again until the response does not decline again.

When the positive reaction begins to decrease, the procedure must be repeated. Repeat this procedure until the condition does not get worse and the individual has improved.

If you do not see any response Repeat the remedy. If there is not a response after three doses the time is now to try a new treatment. Begin again with Step 1.

There is a possibility of taking as much as 6 doses in a day (guideline not included). It's okay to administer greater or lesser than that provided that there is an improvement in the reaction.

The decision to determine the frequency of the administration of homeopathic remedies is comparable as removing a car from of the sand. The driver presses the accelerator, and check if it is sufficient to get you out of the sand. If not, let the accelerator go and allow the car to slide forward. You then press the accelerator once more and check whether the car is moving more forward. The process continues until the car is able to move freely.

Similar to that, you administer your first homeopathic dose, and check the response. It is often enough to get a single dose. If more doses are required it is possible for the person to gain or even worsen and when that happens then you should repeat the dose. It is possible that they will shift a bit more than their first dose before they again stall. Each time they stop or shift a little backwards it is time to repeat the dosage. Follow this energetic rhythm, moving forward as well as slightly backwards until the positive reaction persists and the patient is able to manage any other symptoms their own symptoms.

Administering Remedies to Babies and Toddlers

There are many methods to administer the remedies for infants and toddlers. Just like with all homeopathic treatments choosing the remedy you prefer will be based on your personal preferences. Select the option that is best for you and your dear family members.

Dry Dose

Dry Doses can be used for acute and chronic ailments. Dry Doses are the exact pill.

Make a paste of one or two pills in two spoons of steel until the powder is a consistent consistency. (Using two pills can be simpler for this!). The powder is available using any of these methods. Choose the method that is most effectively for you as well as your child.

(a) The parent dips a their finger clean in powder, and the powdered finger is placed on the tongue of their baby. It is important to ensure that the tablets are covered in powder, especially for babies. The entire powder will not require to be administered only a tiny amount of it can suffice.

OR

(b) (b) A small amount of water could be mixed in with the powdered remedies in a spoon, and then served to the baby.

Liquid Dose

Liquid Doses can be utilized to treat children with tonsillitis or cough that requires an even more powerful response from a treatment. Additionally, when repeated use of the remedy is needed. It is often hard to choose between liquid or dry dosages - both are fine. Always choose to choose the best one for your needs!

4. Place four pills (do not need the need to be broken) within 4 ounces of chilled boiling water. The process can be carried out in bottles for babies or glass/beaker. Wait approx 5 mins.

shake the bottle (or stir the glass or beaker) five times per each dose.

When dispensing bottle for a baby, permit the baby to drink around 5ml' of the liquid (without taking the pills) in each dosage. You can let them drink more than this amount, however, you'll need prepare a brand new bottle in case they consume the bottle in a hurry.

If you are dispensing via a glass or beaker offer the child one teaspoon of the liquid (without pills) to each dosage.

Repeat until a positive reaction is observed. Check out the Dosage Chart within this book.

Be sure that young children as well as children don't consume the pill with the liquid.

Shaking or stirring the remedy is to boost the potency of the remedy. It is also known as "plussing the remedy.

Administering Remedies to Older Children & Adults

Dry Dose

Dry Doses work well for any acute ailment. Dry Doses are the pill in itself.

Begin with one dose.

If a positive reaction is achieved, there's no requirement to repeat the treatment until the response does not get worse.

When the positive reaction begins to decrease, the procedure is to be repeated. Repeat this procedure until the condition does not get worse and the individual is improving.

If there is no response Repeat the remedy. If you still have no reaction after four doses, you are ready to consider a new treatment. Begin again with Step 1.

It is possible to take as many as six doses per every day (this is not a strict rule and the remedies may be prescribed at any time needed once they've created an increase in the reaction).

Liquid Dose

Liquid Doses are suitable by adults and kids who suffer from ailments like cough or tonsillitis that require a more powerful action from the remedy. In addition, frequent repeating of the treatment is needed. It is often difficult to determine between liquid or dry dosages Both are fine. It is best to choose which one works best for your needs!

In an empty glass (or drink bottle) about 300ml. Wait for 5 mins. Pills need not be dissolved prior to administration.

Consume one teaspoonful (or consume the same amount if it is contained in the form of a bottle). Mix 5 times prior to every dosage (or shake the bottle five times prior to each dosage). Tablets need not be dissolved prior to administering.

Repeat the procedure until positive results are observed. Check out the Dosage Chart within this book.

Shaking or stirring the remedy is to boost the potency of the remedy. This is known as "plussing or the remedy. The benefits of plussing are when the individual's overall health and vitality is affected by an severe disease.

Dosage and Frequency

The amount of dosage used will depend upon the severity of each particular instance. The dosage of 30c is appropriate for the majority of acute ailments.

A regular dose is often needed in cases of illness that comes abruptly and then strongly (tonsillitis or fever) as well as less frequent doses can be prescribed for an advancing disease. The dose chart found within this book outlines certain rules.

Once you've given the solution, you need to stop giving the remedy as when you notice an intense positive reaction or an improvement. If you see only one small change, you can continue providing the remedy, however less frequently.

Take up to 3 doses. If you don't see any improvement following this procedure, you've chosen the wrong treatment.

If your symptoms are changing then you should revisit the patient and with changes in symptoms (coughs frequently alter). If the patient is receiving homeopathic medical treatment from a professional, and you're unable to treat the acute issue ask your doctor for assistance if you are able to.

Chapter 9: Which Potency to Use?

There is a wide range of remedies you can utilize in homeopathic treatments. Homeopathic practitioners will use all kinds of remedies based on the specific situation.

To be used for home prescriptions the most effective dosage for purchase is 30c.

Why? 30c has the potency to cause a reaction in the acute problem. It isn't strong enough to trigger a powerful reaction in any chronic illness. It is important to note that the Vital Force (energetic the body) will always deal with the topmost issue. to be used for home prescriptions that is, an acute condition you're dealing with at a specific time. If you have other ongoing chronic ailments, they're not the top priority during acute, therefore any treatment home recommended will be focused upon the current acute.

Dosage Guideline Chart

The dosages listed are suggested which are helpful for those beginning their journey. However, it is best to examine each person separately and administer doses as required.

Illness Severity

Suggested Dosage

Completely Ill:-

A person is totally overwhelmed with their illness. It is possible that they are lying in bed or shivering, and may be very unwell.

Example:

Influenza, Tonsillitis, Virus, Ailment, Pain, Injuries, etc.

Each 30 minute interval until improvements are observed. Space out your time less. Then stop when a positive reaction persists.

Ill:-

The person in pain needs to be relieved and could or not be experiencing the middle of a

Example:

Abscess, cough; stomach Bug and more.

Each 2 hours for a period of time until improvements are observed. After that, space it out more. Then stop when a positive reaction is present.

Less Ill:-

Someone may require a little relief but they can handle with their situation.

Example:

The sore Throat (early phase) or Teething. Head Cold or The Chicken Pox; etc.

Between 4 and six hours. After that, space it out more. End when a strongly positive reaction is maintained.

The symptoms are mild and less severe Less Ill with mild symptoms

The person does not require immediate relief, but usually requires the longer-term assistance rather than treatment

Example:

Anaemia; Exhaustion; Teething; etc.

A daily dose is recommended for a certain duration. Tissue Salts can be a great alternative to 30c potency, and can be found in many grocery stores that sell health food. They're a fantastic choice to take daily doses of support. The selection of salt for the tissue is based upon the individual issue.

Sourcing Your Remedies

The majority of health food stores stock a wide range of remedies that are homeopathic. There are many internet-based pharmacies for homeopathic remedies all over the globe that will deliver remedies right to your door. Follow me on

Facebook and Twitter for my personal tips regarding this.

I would advise you to go to a trusted homeopathic clinic that follows the strictest instructions for how to prepare homeopathic remedies.

It's a great idea to keep a large supply of medicines so you're prepared to respond when someone is poorly. There are many homeopathic pharmacies that offer Remedy Kits, which contain some of the most popular remedies to be used at home for prescribing. There are a myriad of medicines available, however they don't require any prescribing. The solutions listed in this guide should be able to cover the most urgent home prescribing scenarios.

It's not required to have an Remedy Kit. It is possible to build your own collection of cures in time. When you've finished reading the book, make note of the remedies you believe would be beneficial to yourself and those you love Start with the ones you think are needed, and then work your way through those. A remedy kit will always include remedies that you will never utilize, so you should only purchase the Kit when you're certain that this is the remedy you are looking for.

Storing Your Remedies

Place your medicines in a cool, dark and secure area.

There are a myriad of urban legends about homeopathy that have gained a lot of attention over time. A few of them are:

Avoid using remedies that contain smelly substances. No necessity!

Beware of Wi-Fi's remedies. This is not the case!

Keep remedies stored in a form of casing that is protected It is not required!

Avoid taking remedies with food. No!

Mint toothpaste may hinder remedies from working. But not!

It is best to avoid coffee. Absolutely!

Remedies are not able to pass through airport x-ray machines The truth is that they are not! They're distributed across the globe and are delivered safely.

Avoid touching the remedy - If you're taking an herbal remedy on your own, or giving it an individual in your family using the remedy, touching it is acceptable. Of course, you should keep this at a minimum due to safety and health motives. Doing so will not invalidate any remedy.

The homeopathic cures are distributed across the globe and the variety of processes involved in shipping do not negate their value. Coffee and toothpaste do make remedies ineffective - however, if someone is sensitive to coffee or mint, that is an indication of their individual profile.

Acute Ailments

Accidents - Minor (Bumps & Bruises)

Aconite

Most effective treatment to treat shock.
First, if the shock is evident. One dose
should be sufficient (repeat as required).
Distressed, frightened, anxious. Children
may have dilation the look of shock could be
seen on the face. The fear of dying.

Arnica

Abrasions and bumps. to help reduce shock
as well as reduce swelling, and the pain.
Increases the healing process. A person will
frequently say "I'm OK" even though they're
not. It's worse to touch. Helps prevent
bruising. Relief from pain. You can also
apply Arnica cream on top of your skin - just
follow the directions on the packageto apply
it topically. The most common side effect of
Arnica. If one feels emotional "bruised" this
is a great remedy.

Bellis Perennis

Deep bruising. Utilize when Arnica doesn't help, or if the bruising is far into soft tissue. Bellis-perennis provides a special sign of bruising on the breast. If the swelling has subsided but the lump persists.

Bryonia

A painful swelling of the fluid around a injuries or sprains. The worst case scenario is when you is the desire to stay in a completely still position. It is painful to stitch (keynote). The area is hot and red. It's a swollen, red part.

Hypericum

Pain in the nerve. The pain is shooting. The area is inflamed and painful. The areas that are prone to nerves include the finger tips as well as the coccyx. The pain is usually more severe than it seems (eg. pressing your finger against the door of a car and Coccyx).

Ledum

Severe bruising. The strain feels numb and cold that is the primary reason of this cure (sprains and strains are often warmer to the touch, however, if they are cold, think of Ledum). It is better for applications that are cold.

Rhus Tox

As a result of injury or fall. The swelling, stiffness, and pain. The tendons and joints of the larger joints are strained. tendon. The most effective treatment for injuries sustained in sports. Inflammation and redness are commonly noticed. The feeling of being restless is the main feature for Rhus Tox physical or psychologically.

Ruta

In constant pain, bruising and inability to walk. The ligaments and tendons are smaller (wrists as well as ankles). They are more prone to damage from pressure, sitting, or walking. It is often used in conjunction when combined with Rhus Tox, particularly to treat sports-related injuries.

Make sure you consult your doctor following an injury or accident.

Aches & Pains

Arnica

All-round pain relief. Achy and bruised. Can't get comfortable. Muscular discomfort.

Bryonia

Stiffness and extreme stitching discomfort (keynote stitching pain). Irritable. The worst thing is that you is prone to lying totally still.

Hypericum

Great remedy for injuries or pain in the nerve. Excellent for injuries to spinal cord and coccyx. Sciatica and feeling of nerves that are pinched. The pain is sharp, pulsing and intense.

Kali-Carb

The most common treatment to treat back pain is. Most often, the lower back. The back feels stiff and weak. The back aches like it's fractured. It is difficult to get into bed during the late at night.

Nux Vomica

Spasms. The pain is sudden and sharp at the moment of you turn. The sensation is cold. More comfortable with warmer temperatures. Impatient and irritable with the pain. Most often, it is due to overwork or living too much.

Rhus Tox

A great remedy for muscle pain or injury. It is stiff when the first time you move. It then becomes looser (Keynote). Restless both physically as well as mentally. The best option is heat, specifically a warm baths.

Ruta

Similar to Rhus Tox. Tendon pain. Itchy and painful rheumatic symptoms. The pain is less if you lie in a position. Stressed about injuries or pain. Most often, it is caused by excessive use or injuries from sports.

AnxiETY / NERVous

Aconite

Excellent remedy for anxiety and anxiety about events to come (such such as exams, speech or any other special event). Afraid and stressed. Feeling panicked or in anxiety. Palpitations.

Arg-Nit

The most common treatment for anxiety-related anticipatory. Nervous and concerned about an future events. Diarrhoea and loose stools, with"nerves". Restless and anxious. Stressing over the 'What Ifs' that may not happen. Wanting sweet, sugary foods.

Arsenicum

Common remedy for anxiety and general stress. Nerves and anxieties are a common occurrence as well as a great deal of anxiety and agitation. Strives to get everything perfect and organized. They can be very exigent. A fear of their own wellbeing. Also, anxiety about their health and well-being of loved ones (children and old family members). Despair. The fear of dying, sickness and serious illness. The most aggravating time is around 1 am. It is a time of nervousness, anxiety and tension.

Gelsemium

Another popular remedy. More frequent urination "nerves" and a feeling of better when you urinate. It goes into freeze mode. The thoughts go to empty. Stuttering or shaking with nerves. Legs are jittery and weak.

Kali-phos

Nerve "tonic". Anxiety, nervousness, and dread with no explanation. Gloomy. The brain fag.

Lycopodium

Low self-confidence, and a lack of self-esteem, despite the fact that they're extremely competent. They will be well-prepared to face the next challenge and, despite the fact that they believe they're inadequate, they'll end up being awe-inspiring when they begin. The nerves will ease once they start. Constipation and a loud "gas".

Black Eye

Attention medical attention is needed. It is possible to administer homeopathy along with.

Arnica

Eyeball bruises. In case of shock, it can help reduce the pain and swelling. It speeds up the healing process. People will frequently claim that "I'm OK" even though they're not. The worst thing to do is touching. It prevents bruises. Relief from pain.

Ledum

The most common treatment for black eyes. If Arnica was prescribed, but there is still bruising take a look at Ledum.

Symphytum

Eyeball pain that is severe that is swollen and red. If Arnica was prescribed, and swelling is gone, but irritation persists, you should consider Symphytum. (Symphytum is typically considered to be a treatment to treat fractures, however bones are not required to be broken or fractured for it to be thought of.)

Chapter 10: Broken Bones / Fractures

Attention medical attention is needed. Homeopathy is a treatment option that can be administered in conjunction with.

Aconite

This can be done if shock occurs.

Arnica

to help reduce shock and reduce swelling as well as discomfort. It speeds up the healing process. A person will frequently say "I'm OK" even though they're not. The worst thing is touching - actually, it's a pain. It prevents bruises. It also helps relieve pain. It is believed that bruising is the primary ingredient of Arnica. If one feels emotional "bruised" this is a great remedy.

Bryonia

It is recommended to treat it If there is a lot of pain, and movement becomes painful. Pain from stitching (keynote). Hold the painful area in order to hold it there. The worst thing for movement is that it you will be tempted to lay completely in a slumber.

Symphytum

Primary remedy for assisting in healing of fractured bone and broken fractures. It eases pain and speed up the healing process of fractured and broken bones. Utilize after bone has been placed.

Symphytum is a good choice to support the body in the period it takes for an injury or fracture to heal. The dosage can range from 30c to 60c but it's best to choose a lesser potency of 6c for this situation. This permits a daily treatment to be administered.

Burns & Scalds - Minor

Notification medical attention is needed. Homeopathy is a treatment option that can be administered in conjunction with.

The burns may affect only a small area however they can be intensely pain-inducing. The treatment of severe burns must be done with respect, and a professional in burns and medical treatment should be arranged immediately.

Aconite

This can be done if shock occurs.

Arnica

To relieve pain and reduce inflammation. Additionally, it helps with the effects of shock.

Arsenicum

Pains that burn. Accompanying blisters. Better for heat.

Belladonna

There is a lot of redness and heat however no damage to the skin. Throbbing pain.

Cantharis

The most common treatment for minor burns, scalds and burns. Blisters and pain. Better for cold compresses.

Causticum

The pain is burning. Blisters. Help with soreness on the area of previous burns. If Cantharis doesn't help then you should consider Causticum.

Chickenpox

Ant-tart

The pustules are slowly appearing. Cough with a rattling chest and difficulty in coughing out mucus. The person is agitated and whimpering, angry. The tongue is white and coated. Nausea and dizziness.

Merc Sol / Merc-Viv

Pustules that begin to release pus, then turn yellow. The digestion may be affected by the appearance of slimy green stools. The worst is in the evening. The itch is worse when you are warm in mattress. Moist eruptions.

Pulsatilla

The symptoms of chickenpox can be emotional - whining, crying, does not like being isolated, seeks comfort. The symptoms can vary and a child may want to breathe in fresh air and feel better due to it.

Rhus Tox

A common treatment for chickenpox is to use a steroid. The sting is itchy, painful and irritating. Itching that is intense and pustule-like. can be worse when scratched and more severe at night. Itching can be improved with hot waters. Expansions all over the body. Unrestful and difficult to sleep.

Sulphur

Itchy, red, and itchy. The healing process for chickenpox is slow and may recur. The itch is more severe in hot temperatures especially the heat of the mattress. When scratched, skin gets burned.

Colds

Aconite

The first signs appear, especially following exposure to cold. Itchy, coughing burning, and a rawness in the tongue, more so in a stuffy environment. A thirst for cool drinking water. Anxious. Eyes dilate. They can also have high temperatures. A fear of dying.

Arsenicum

The discharge is watery and burning. It causes the lip to be sensitive. Frequent painful sneezing. Eyes are burning. Sinuses blocked, painful. Pains that burn. Aching. It was filled with food at night. A cold and thirsty feeling. Very anxious and restless. Irritable. It's thirsty when you drink a glass of water.

Belladonna

Sudden, violent onset. Extremely hot. It can start because from being cold. It can cause burning, shivering and a rawness of ears, throat and the nose. Thirsty. A dry, warm body. The feet are cold. Thirstless.

Bryonia

The signs appear slowly. The thirsty can be triggered by large quantities of water that is cold. Every movement can make them more uncomfortable. Are you looking to just "bear with a sore neck Headache.

Ferr-phos

The first phase of cold. Sore throats, colds, and colds quickly. Watery discharge, blood streaked. Nosebleeds. There are no other signs. Mucousy the throat. Hoarse. Throbbing headache.

Hepar Sulph

The cold is watery and turns into the thick green and yellow mucous. Draughts and colds are a pet peeve. People will need to get warm, and be angry as well as impatient and critical. Insensitive to the sensation of pain. Nasal drips down the back of throat. Smell may disappear.

Kali-mur

Common head colds that are stuffy and are accompanied by ear infections. The ears feel stuffed and irritable. the head. A white discharge that comes from the nose. The backside of the tongue is covered with a white-colored tongue.

Merc Sol / Merc-Viv

The eyes, the ears and the throat can be affected. It starts as a cold that is watery the mucous then turns green and yellow and can cause irritation of the skin around the lips and nose. The tongue gets coated, in a sour taste. The mouth musty. The saliva is swollen and the sweating. More severe in the late at night. A blocked painful sinus. It's a hot day, and so are moods! Thirsty. Sweating.

Nat Mur

A lot of sniffing and sneezing. Runny nose. Thirsty. Lips are dry and swollen. A watery discharge from the eyes or nose.

Nux Vom

Nose can feel constricting, headache and constipation. It is also irritable throughout the day, and is it is blocked in the evening. Watery discharge. Sneezing frequently. Cold. Irritable. Bossy. Extremely hot. Sweating. The snuffles of babies.

Phosphorous

Blood streaked discharge. Profuse discharge. Hoarse. Itchy throat. An increase in appetite. Extremely thirsty for cold beverages. Desires ice-cream. It is possible that they are not as sick as fever would suggest children are often joyfully. Enjoys being with family and can be easily trusted. Aversion to dark, ghosts or violent storms. Better for short naps. The cold can quickly reach the chest.

Pulsatilla

Smell and taste impaired. A thick, yellow-green and bland discharge. The symptoms are more severe during the evening, or inside however, they feel better outside in fresh air. The cough can develop. Children can be emotional or clingy, and may feel sorry for their own. Whiny. Thirstless.

Coldsores

Nat Mur

The most common remedy to treat the cold sores (acutely). Lip sores and the area around the mouth. Lips are dry and cracked.

Rhus Tox

Mundus and chin sores. Itching and burning. The taste of your mouth is bitter.

Sepia

Lip sores. Sometimes, they are linked with hormonal fluctuations.

Cold sores that recur are best addressed by an herbalist.

Conjunctivitis

Apis

A stinging red and puffy eyes. Eyes roiling hot with tears. Painful. It is better for cold-based applications.

Arg-Nit

Eyes are red and inflamed. Eyelids joined. A sensitivity to the light. There is a lot of smelly yellow discharge.

Arsenicum

Eyes are burning. Eyes sensitized to light, and burning.

Belladonna

Eyes are very red, inflamed and dry. Pupils dilated. The pupils are sensitive to lights.

Euphrasia

Excellent remedy for any eyes problem. Eyes that are swollen, burning and itchy. Many and many blinks. Eyes constantly dry and burning on the skin's surface. Eyes feel like sand. The eyes are filled with pus.

Pulsatilla

The most common treatment for conjunctivitis. Eyes hurt, sore and itchy. The discharge is thick and yellow (Important it does not harm the skin's outer surface). Eyelids are glued. The Pulsatilla photo can be observed as clingy and wailing.

Silica

Yellow discharge. Eyes are sore. Inflamed tear duct or blocked.

Sulphur

Hot, painful, red eye irritation, burning, red. The sensation of grit or sand in the eyes. Itchy. The irritation that eyes get from washing can be worse. This sensation of heat is the most important thing to Sulphur.

Constipation (Acute)

This treatment is meant for immediate use only. If constipation continues it is recommended to consult a homoeopathic doctor for the selection of appropriate treatment.

Calc-carb

A great remedy for constipation. Children aren't really concerned by constipation. It is quite large and tough and may be light in shade. The child is generally easygoing, but may be stubborn.

Causticum

Stool hard to get rid of. The texture may be softer or covered with mucous. Crampy, colicky pains. The stool is easier to pass if you stand. Children who are extremely sensitive and are not averse to the injustice.

Lycopodium

The stomach is bloated and full of gas. There is a lot of flatulence. It feel better with wind. Stools hard, knotty. Sometimes they feel they're not enough although they're very competent.

Mag Mur

Constipation due to milk. Strenuous effort to move stool, but it doesn't happen. Stools were passed through with difficulty, and are shaped like small balls. The pain of ramming. He is anxious and doesn't like conflict.

Nat Mur

The stool is being passed through, however it doesn't happen. Once stool appears the person feels there's some more work to do. They can appear small and breaking. People tend to be shy who are able to keep their emotions in check.

Nux Vomica

A constant urge to pass stool, but not much or nothing happens. It feels like there's left to be passed. It can occur in conjunction with diarrhoea. The stool is large and hard.

You may have overindulged at the party, or at a restaurant and so on. Extremely irritable and difficult to accept.

Silica

Stool is a difficult thing to get rid of. The child will be grunting and screaming for it to be removed. Stool could be removed partially and then disappear. Can burn afterwards. Children can be fragile, yet also very self-confident within their own.

Coughs

Treatment- This can be used for emergency prescribing only. If you are suffering from persistent cough the homoeopathic consultation might be needed to determine the optimal remedies that match.

Aconite

Dry, hard, loud, barking, cough. Sometimes, it happens suddenly following a shock or a fear that is emotional (weather) or psychological. The exposure to cold wind can be the trigger. Midnight is an important hour. Constant. Irritating. More so in the evening. It could be high temperature.

Ant-tart

Simple remedy for spotting. A loose rattling cough. A difficult rattling breath. It is possible to hear the rattling within the chest. The larynx is tickling, which can aggravate the cough. A lot of phlegm. Phlegm coughing can give some relief. It is possible to gasp and yawn. cough.

Belladonna

Sudden onset. Extremely hot. A dry, twitching, intense cough, and headache. A swollen face. The child may be crying to prepare for the difficult cough. Vocals are choppy. Sharp pain in chest.

Bryonia

Slowly increasing in severity. It is a painful and dry hacking cough. The person holds their chest, side or even the head as they cough. The person is thirsty and needs a lot of fluid. Would like to be with a friend and be at a distance. Breathlessness is aggravating. The coughing fits. Disturbs sleep. Itchy, irritating cough. It is better to lie on a the side that is painful. Dry cough, minimal or no anticipation. Thirsty. Extremely irritable moods.

Calc-carb

Dry, tickly cough in the evening and at night, dry cough early in the morning. More likely in humid weather or windy days.

Drosera

The big cough treatment. A violent, constant cough. The cough is agitated, spasmodic, including gagging, retching and vomiting. More severe at night, when lying down. Use hands to hold the chest and cough. A great remedy for whooping cough. Most often, it starts with a tickle on the in the throat.

Ferr-phos

Dry cough that is short and tickly. It is dry and hard itchy to the cough. The cough is usually a recurring issue in the evening. A good treatment when there are only a few distinct symptoms.

Hepar-sulph

A rattly and loose, deep chesty cough. Chesty and Phlegmy. Difficult expectoration. Phlegm is yellow and thick (same as mucous that comes from the nose). It is important to be aware that a cough may occasionally become dry and croupy. It is worse when cold is present or covered - would like to be kept warm. Impatient, anxious and irritable. Could have a high-temperature. Bedtime sets off cough.

Ignatia

Cough that follows an emotional incident (grief anger, disagreement, abuse and abuse, or bullying). Dry and hollow, spasmodic cough. The more often they cough, the more severe the condition gets.

Ipecac

Chesty cough: moist, sounds of wheezy rattling, usually without any phlegm. It sounds like a wheezy cough. It is difficult to expectorate. The typical cough is followed by vomiting or gags. Sometimes, it can lead to nosebleeds.

Kali-bich

The cough is rumbling and causes sinus issues. A lot of stringy, thick discharge that can be difficult to eliminate. The best remedy for sinus troubles.

Kali-carb

Dry, hard-choking cough. It is worse between 2 and 4 am. Cough that is painful. Constant cough that wakes the child. It may end with a gagging attack or vomiting. The tendency to contract colds.

Phosphorous

Great all-round lung remedy. Dry, hard and tickly cough. A tickling cough that is felt in the larynx the chest and throat. The cough can be unsteady. The chest is tight and it is like there's a feeling of pressing on it. It is worse when you are talking, laughing or moving from warm to cool air. The worst is in the evenings, specifically after sunset. Blood from the mucous streaked. Colds that reach the chest. Chronic coughs. Most often, it is linked with an susceptibility or history of asthma or chest infections. Children wake up at late at night. You must sit to cough. Feels thirsty for water and ice cold drinks. Likes ice cream.

Pulsatilla

Dry cough that is yellow/green in mucus or phlegm. Also, it can be chesty. The worst time to experience chesty is in the morning, evening or lying in a the warm space. A person wants fresh air but does not feel hungry or thirsty. Clingy, teary and extremely clingy. Thirstless. A loud, rattling breath. Phlegm is difficult to expel It may also taste unpleasant. Keynotes on Pulsatilla are dry and clingy.

Rhus Tox

Dry and irritated cough. Worse after getting wet. A bit agitated.

Rumex

Dry, hacking cough. Incessant tickle of the throat and larynx. Continuous cough that disturbs the sleep. Caused by changes in temperatures of the air, such as switching rooms, opening the fridge or refrigerator, and dropping temperature at evening. The breath of cold or cool air can cause. The burning sensation and redness of the chest.

Spongia

The best remedy to treat coughs! The dry barking of the croupy cough can be heard as if a seal is dogs barking. The sound of breathing is whirling when you breathe. The worst thing is at night. It is better to eat, drink and steam. A feeling of something happening in the larynx or throat awakes at midnight, then wakes abruptly. More severe in the morning and during the thrill. Crupy cough. The attack of coughing. Keynotes refer to coughs that can be dry and, sometimes, barking.

Croup

Aconite

Initial stage. It appears suddenly. Often around midnight. The barking, hard, dry cough. Constant. Irritating. There may be high temperatures.

Hepar-sulph

Crying, coughing. The cough is loose and rumbling. It is difficult to cough up phlegm. It coughs up thick yellow Phlegm. It is extremely cold and needs to be protected. Impatient, impatient and critical when coughing.

Phosphorous

Dry, tickling cough. It gets worse when you breathe conversations, cold air or laughing. A burning, dry sensation that is felt in the throat. Hoarseness. Cough that lingers. You're thirsty and would like ice-cold beverages or ice cream.

Spongia

The most commonly-used cure. A dry, croupy cough that barks is like hearing a seal barking. A typical the sound of a croup. The coughing sounds are typical. The Spongia virus should be at the top of your list when it comes to Croup.